The Medical Student Career Handbook

The Medical Student Career Handbook

SECOND EDITION

Edited by

ELIZABETH COTTRELL

Year 1 Academic Specialty Trainee in General Practice

First edition also edited by

CHRISTELE REBORA & MARK WILLIAMS

Radcliffe Publishing
Oxford • New York

Radcliffe Publishing Ltd
18 Marcham Road
Abingdon
Oxon OX14 1AA
United Kingdom

www.radcliffe-oxford.com
Electronic catalogue and worldwide online ordering facility.

British Library Cataloguing in Publication Data

A catalogue record for this book is available from the British Library.

ISBN-13 978 1 84619 304 0

Typeset by Pindar NZ, Auckland, New Zealand
Printed and bound by TJI Digital, Padstow, Cornwall, UK

Contents

Foreword to the first edition   viii

Preface to the second edition   ix

About the editor   x

Contributors to the second edition   xi

Acknowledgements   xii

General career topics

1 Introduction   1

2 Experiences of others   4

3 Career development toolkit   8

4 Preparation for future jobs   21

5 Career support, advisers and fairs   31

6 Mentors and educational supervisors   41

7 What is good about a career in medicine?   47

8 Medical career pathways   50

9 The Foundation Programme   58

Medical student topics

10 Broadening your clinical experience   64

11 Application to Foundation Programme posts   78

12 The consolidation period   87

Postgraduate topics

13 Postgraduate working conditions and pay   90

14 Specialty training   99

15 Specialty profiles   107

16 Academic medicine: incorporating research and medical
education into your career   126

17 GPs with a special interest   133

18 Working abroad   136

19 Diverse medical careers   141

20 What else can I do with a degree in medicine?   146

Support

21 Societies and organisations   149

22 Discrimination and how to avoid it   157

Appendix 1   164

Appendix 2   169

Appendix 3   170

Appendix 4   171

Appendix 5   172

Appendix 6   173

Appendix 7   175

Index   177

A partnership between Keele University, the University of Warwick, the University of Birmingham and the West Midlands Deanery

UNIVERSITY^{OF} BIRMINGHAM

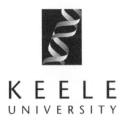

KEELE
UNIVERSITY

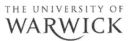

NHS
West Midlands

Foreword to the first edition

I am delighted to write the foreword for this excellent book, whose arrival is timely given the introduction of new foundation and specialist training programmes across the United Kingdom.

The recent changes proposed in *Modernising Medical Careers* underline the importance of the benefits of informed career choice, not only in terms of efficient training programmes now, but also for the future generations of doctors. It is very likely that this will have added significance for those beginning a medical career later in life through the increasing number of UK-based graduate entry programmes at medical school, or for medical graduates entering the NHS from Europe or from other parts of the world.

This book complements the UK-wide approach to the delivery of career management initiatives that was launched as part of the Department of Health's *Modernising Medical Careers* strategy. As Chair of the working group that produced the national careers management strategy, I warmly welcome this book.

A key feature is that it has been researched and written by consumers; by final year medical students with contributions and support from more experienced consultants and general practitioners. I believe that it provides a superb source of information and focused help for medical students and junior doctors that will help them prepare effectively for their foundation programmes and for specialist training. It will also provide a valuable resource for educational supervisors, GP trainers and clinical tutors. I commend it to you.

Professor Steve Field
Postgraduate Dean, West Midlands
Chair, UK Modernising Medical Careers Advisory Board
July 2006

Preface to the second edition

Following the success of the first edition and the multiple changes to medical careers in a short space of time, a revision of *The Medical Student Career Handbook* was essential. The original concept of the *Handbook* was that its development and content was medical student led. As I have been lucky enough to not only graduate, but also successfully complete my Foundation Programme and embark on academic general practice training, I was keen to involve current medical students in this revision. I therefore invited medical students from the West Midlands Workforce Deanery to advise me on the aspects of the first edition they found helpful, those they thought required changing and information or guidance that had previously been omitted. What has followed has been an improvement to and an update of the first edition.

Writing about medical careers is littered with difficulties, especially in today's climate of frequent change and much controversy. It is an exciting time as many changes are afoot, all with the aim of making both training and the NHS as a whole much improved and designed to meet modern healthcare needs. I therefore make no apology that some information in this book will go out of date; this is merely a reflection of the speed with which things are changing. However, I can assure you that much of the advice and support provided within the *Handbook* is generic and will be long-standing for medical students and Foundation trainees over the early years of their medical careers.

In addition to the acknowledgements I make subsequently, I would also like to thank the staff with whom I have closely worked in both the West Midlands Workforce Deanery and Keele University School of Medicine and who have provided much support and encouragement in my personal goals to improve career support at a wider level for both medical students and junior doctors. I really could not do anything on my own and I am thankful for them allowing me to make a small contribution towards a greater end and for informing the work that I have undertaken to date. I would also like to thank the Keele Medical Student Career Committee (KMSCC) for their hard work and dedication towards providing additional career support for Keele medical students. In addition, the insights that the KMSCC have provided have been invaluable in highlighting the needs of medical students regarding career support.

Lizzie Cottrell
Year 1 Academic Specialty Trainee in General Practice
January 2009

About the editor

Elizabeth Cottrell worked hard during her training to gain a broad knowledge and experience base. Her aim has always been to be a general practitioner (GP), and latterly an 'academic GP', but she is a firm believer in keeping career options open during medical school. As a result of this her work has been varied. In contrast to her time spent at a high-security forensic psychiatry hospital, she has assisted paediatric diabetes specialist nurses to gain funding for a nurse prescribing course and has been involved in laboratory research, which has discovered some potentially exciting results. In addition to clinical training, Elizabeth is currently in the process of undertaking a Masters in Medical Science and musculoskeletal-based research. She has experienced medicine from perspectives other than those of doctors, through nearly five years' part-time work as a healthcare assistant on orthopaedic and medical wards, a summariser of notes in a GP practice and as a hospital domestic earlier on in her career.

Contributors to the second edition

Abigail Gee BSc(Hons) PhD, Warwick Medical School

Angela Nelmes, student at Keele University School of Medicine

Anna Sutherland, studied at Keele University School of Medicine

Antony Sarno, student at Keele University School of Medicine

Charlene Binding, Career Management Associate at Trent Multi-Professional Deanery

Cheryl Bennet, student at Keele University School of Medicine

David Metcalf BSc(Hons), Warwick Medical School

Emma Stephens, student at Keele University School of Medicine

Helen Goodyear, West Midlands Workforce Deanery Head of Postgraduate School of Paediatrics and Associate Postgraduate Dean for Flexible Training

Hinesh Patel, student at Keele University School of Medicine

Margaret Lawless, senior human resources adviser and a recruitment consultant

Naomi Tyrrell studied at Warwick Medical School

Patrick Daly studied at Warwick Medical School

Ruby Baig, student at Keele University School of Medicine

Ruth Chambers, Professor of Primary Care at Staffordshire University

Sarah Kinsman BSc(Hons), student at Warwick Medical School

Sarah Peacock BSc(Hons), student at Warwick Medical School

Stephanie Triance studied at Warwick Medical School

Acknowledgements

As a result of the nature of the content of this handbook, some content has been derived from key documents. Any use of such documents has been fully referenced. This second edition has been built from the foundations laid by the first, therefore I would like to, once again, acknowledge the work of the people who helped with the first edition.

First we must sincerely thank Professor Steve Field, without whom the first edition of this book would not have been possible. We would also like to thank Steve for writing the foreword of the first edition.

It is with thanks that we acknowledge that we initially followed in the footsteps of the work the East Midlands Healthcare Workforce Deanery laid down with regards to career information for medical students. The East Midlands Healthcare Workforce Deanery and the University of Nottingham first produced a *Nottingham Medical School Career Handbook* and has since produced multiple revisions. Through recognising how worthwhile a document such as this is, we felt that a book containing such important information should be available to all medical students and junior doctors. We welcomed the input and experience of Charlene Binding, who assisted in the development of the first edition of this book.

We should like to sincerely thank all people who participated in surveys that enabled us to compile the *specialty profiles* and *experiences of others*.

Thanks also to those people who approached and 'chased' doctors to help us obtain all the specialty profiles. They are: Charlene Kennedy (Manchester School of Medicine); Nathalie Rebora (St George's International Medical School) and Jenny Robertson (Newcastle upon Tyne Medical School).

We should like to thank the following professionals for critiquing sections and chapters of the first edition of this book: Dr Maggie Allen, Mr Mohamed Arafa, Dr Colin Campbell, Mr Paul Deemer, Dr Rose Johnson, Mrs Janet Monkman and Mr Manjit Obhrai.

Thank you to the following people for their additional input to the first edition: Mrs Clare Kennedy who was the Careers Project Manager for the West Midlands Deanery; Dr Chris Nancollas, GP; and Helen Westall who studied at Barts and the London medical school and was the 2005 Trauma Conference Organiser.

Most of the illustrations used throughout the book were designed and drawn by Elizabeth Cottrell.

Introduction

In order to have a fulfilled and enjoyable career, you need to make decisions that are right for you. Not only this, but medical career pathways and application processes can change, sometimes with less than one year's notice, so you need to be prepared and equipped with the skills to handle whatever is thrown at you. This book will introduce you to the key skills, resources and support that will help you to have a successful medical career.

At graduation, over half of new doctors do not know what specialty they want to enter[1] and many subsequently change career direction. In addition, 55% of doctors report that they are quite or very dissatisfied with the career advice and guidance they have received. Furthermore, 17% say a lack of advice led them to making decisions in their training that they now regret.[2] The British Medical Association's 2008 report from *The Cohort Study of 2006 Medical Graduates* revealed the following career-related findings from doctors just over a year after graduation:[3]

- about 50% of doctors would prefer a career in hospital medicine – the most popular choices being general medicine and surgery
- roughly a quarter of doctors would prefer a career in general practice
- around 20% are undecided about their preferred career path and ultimate career goal
- half had changed their career intentions due to their Foundation Year 1 placements
- the most common causes for change of career intention were work conditions, hours of work and career and promotion prospects
- the majority of doctors reported that careers advice and support was available and, of those, the majority stated it was useful. The main sources of support were careers advisers, clinical tutors, senior colleagues, deanery, the Internet, royal colleges and the British Medical Association/British Medical Journal
- only 4% of doctors were confident that they will get a job in their chosen specialty once their training is complete.

This *Handbook* aims to give you, as medical students and junior doctors, the tools you need to start making your own informed career decisions.

As a result of changes in career structures and initiatives such as Modernising Medical Careers (MMC) doctors are required to have a pro-active and informed approach to career development. Medical students and doctors have to make career decisions early as Specialty Training applications take place less than two years after graduation from medical school; therefore you must start thinking about your future medical career while you are still a student. Improving the quality of career information, advice and counselling is vital if the MMC (and subsequent) reforms and postgraduate training programmes are to be successful.

No one can make career decisions for you. You have to learn how to help yourself to make informed career choices. This *Handbook* gives you help, tips, advice and signposts for further guidance for embarking on a successful and personally appropriate career.

BOX 1.1

Why should you read this handbook?
● There is less time to make career decisions than you think.
● It will alert you to the facilities and resources that are available.
● It is a source of reliable and consistent information to help you make an informed decision.
● It gives application advice and help with CVs.
● It contains specialty profiles and job statistics.
● It helps you discover your personality type and, therefore, which specialty may suit you.
● It informs you of the career advice and support available and how to access these.
● It alerts you to ongoing medical career changes under the MMC initiative.
● It is an interactive resource full of ideas and support for early career development and will be useful right through your junior doctor (Foundation) years – so keep it safe!

Useful texts and websites containing information about career development and useful contact details can be found at the end of each chapter and in Appendix 1. The web addresses provided were correct, and in use, at the time of writing.

REFERENCES

1 Anderson C and Binding C. *Nottingham Medical School Career Handbook.* 2nd ed. Nottingham: Trent Postgraduate Deanery and the University of Nottingham; 2005.
2 Jackson C, Ball J and Hirsh W. *Informing Choices: the need for career advice in medical training.* Cambridge: National Institute for Careers Education and Counselling; 2004.
3 British Medical Association Health Policy & Economic Research Unit. *Cohort Study 2006 Medical Graduates Second Report.* London: BMA; 2008.

FURTHER READING

Agha R. *Making Sense of Your Medical Career: your strategic guide to success*. London: Hodder Education; 2005.

Blundell A, Harrison R and Turney B. *The Essential Guide to Becoming a Doctor*. London: BMJ Publishing Group; 2004.

British Medical Association. *Becoming a Doctor: entry in 2009*. 9th ed. London: BMA Board of Science and Education; 2008.

Eccles S and Ward C. *So You Want to Be a Brain Surgeon*. 2nd revised ed. Oxford: Oxford University Press; 2001.

Elton C and Reid J. *The ROADS to Success*. 2nd ed. Postgraduate Deanery for Kent, Sussex and Surrey; 2008.

Medical Careers Society and Careers Advisory Group. *Nottingham Medical School Career Handbook*. 5th ed. Nottingham: The University of Nottingham and East Midlands Healthcare Workforce Deanery; 2008.

Postgraduate Medical Education and Training Board. *National survey of trainees 2007 summary report*. London: Postgraduate Medical Education and Training Board. Available at: www.pmetb.org.uk/fileadmin/user/QA/Trainee_Survey/National_Survey_of_Trainees_2007_Summary_Report_20080723-Final.pdf (accessed 8 January 2009).

Shakur R. *A Career in Medicine: do you have what it takes?* 2nd ed. London: Royal Society of Medicine; 2006.

2

Experiences of others

Career pathways are different for everyone. This chapter contains information, lessons and advice from people at various stages of their career.

Below are a few experiences of career development from people at various stages of the medical career pathway. Read and reflect on these experiences and see how you can use them to further your career and make appropriate decisions that suit your circumstances. Compare your own experiences with the ones below. Use the comparison constructively to assess how you have got to where you are and to think about avenues you have not considered previously.

Name: Dr Carol Gray

Position: A&E Consultant; Clinical Dean of Undergraduate Medicine, Keele University

Year of graduation: 1982

University of graduation: University of London (Barts)

Highlights of your career: My present job combination takes a lot of beating, although permanent exhaustion is a drawback!

Problems with career development decisions/bad advice: As a junior doctor I struggled with my primary surgical exams. I went to the surgeon appointed by the college for career advice. After listening to me he suggested I give up and also clearly stated that he felt women who did surgery were frustrated singletons. 'At least you are married' was his comment on seeing my wedding ring. Needless to say, I ignored him and achieved my FRCS (A&E) a couple of years later.

Advice to students about career development: Be realistic. Try to find a career path that really excites you (it helps on bad days) but think about what you want out of the rest of your life as well. If you need time off to study, take it. A short period of locums will not hurt and without exams you will not progress. Be honest at job interviews – it usually pays off. Think about how you will feel when you are finally trained and doing the job day after day – it is very different from being a trainee. Also, develop your non-clinical medical skills. My job is about one-third medical education and the rest as an NHS clinician and I think that, increasingly, this is a model for the future, whether education, research, management or other activities are your 'thing'. A change is frequently as good as a rest!

Name: Dr Sharon Turner

Position: GP

Year of graduation: 1986

University of graduation: Birmingham University

Highlights of your career: Family medicine programme, Illawarra Health Authority, NSW, Australia. Joining current practice; becoming a trainer.

Problems with career development decisions/bad advice: I do not remember getting any bad advice.

Good advice received: Work part-time if you can when children are small and do not take long breaks.

Advice to students about career development: Be open-minded. Try and get a broad experience at junior level. Consider working abroad.

Name: Dr Graham Heyes

Position: Senior House Officer

Year of graduation: 2001

University of graduation: University of Manchester

Highlights of your career: Trauma surgery elective in Montreal General Hospital; A&E six-month Senior House Officer (SHO) post at North Staffordshire General Hospital.

Problems with career development decisions/bad advice: The problem-based learning course seems to make it very difficult to pass the MRCP. Hardly anyone in my year has, so far, managed to pass it yet. Going to St Andrews seems to be beneficial to passing the MRCP, a postgraduate exam for those specialising in the medical field. I have had to virtually restart learning medicine (by learning lists as for conventional courses) to enable me to make any headway with passing the exams.

Good advice received: Do some A&E as it gives you confidence about discharging and admitting patients, although it can be stressful at the time and can impair your social life. Buy a house as soon as you can near a hospital. You can always rent it out later.

Advice to students about career development: Better to delay your choice about SHO rotation (surgery, medicine, anaesthesia) until you are sure, rather than getting on a path that you are unsure about.

Name: Dr Fady Magdy

Position: Foundation Year 1 (F1)

Year of graduation: 2005

University of graduation: University of Manchester

Highlights of your career: None stated.

Problems with career development decisions/bad advice: Never had any problems. I knew early on which specialty I wanted to pursue and so I have tailored my under-graduate experience and projects to suit this. I have also chosen suitable rotations for my F1 to gain experience in related specialties.

Good advice received: I received excellent advice from my educational supervisor regarding the experience necessary.

Advice to students about career development: *Be pro-active.* Ask advice from various consultants.

Name: Dr Anna Sutherland

Position: Foundation Year 1 (F1)

Year of Graduation: 2008

University of Graduation: St Andrews / Manchester (based at Keele)

Highlights of your career: Saving a child who was choking and knowing in that moment that medicine really was for me.

Problems with career development decisions/ bad advice: In the nature of the new system we all have to decide on our specialities earlier than before. If you do know what you want early on, don't be afraid to start tailoring your CV towards it. You'll need it sooner than you think.

Good advice received: Be proactive. Try specialities out whenever you get the chance.

Advice to students about career development: Read this book! Really look at who you are and what you want before you decide on your career path.

Name: Mr Ravin Ramtohal

Position: Final year medical student

Year of graduation: 2006

University of graduation: Southampton University Medical School

Highlights of your career: Founding the Southampton medics squash club. I par-ticularly enjoyed the third- and fourth-year attachments, especially dermatology, orthopaedics and ophthalmology.

Problems with career development decisions/ bad advice: Applying for F1 positions was particularly difficult without help from the university.

Good advice received: Third-year pastoral tutor is excellent in her advice in dealing with the pressures of the course.

Advice to students about career development: Build your portfolio and CV, especially aspects that include teamwork and leadership skills.

Name: Emma Stephens

Position: Fourth year medical student

Year of Graduation: 2010

University of Graduation: Keele University

Highlights of your career: Being involved in e-mentoring with brightjournals, being president of the ActiVE society in my second year and being involved with Keele Medical Student Career Committee throughout my second and third years.

Problems with career development decisions/ bad advice: I have a problem with my spine and I have had to think hard about which career path is realistically going to be the best for me to follow. Luckily I have had lots of support and haven't had any bad advice.

Good advice received: Be honest with yourself and accept any limitations that you have and work with them.

Advice to students about career development: Get involved with extra-curricular activities as early on in medical school as you can. They provide you with lots of skills that will be valuable in the future. Also actively seek out support with career decisions – there are lots of people willing to help if you ask!

3

Career development toolkit

This book has been designed to give you the information and skills required to make career decisions and to succeed in the career path you choose. This chapter explicitly provides you with sources of these. The information provided here will assist you in making early career decisions and explain further how to use this book.

ADVICE FOR MANAGING YOUR CAREER DEVELOPMENT

You may not have thought much about your career. However, it is never too soon to start doing something about it.

The most important thing you can do is to be pro-active; your career will not just happen. To be successful in developing a career plan we advise you to:
- listen to others you are working with
- not be afraid to ask questions, people are generally very happy to talk about their jobs
- take career development opportunities
- seek out help when required
- ask your university if you would like the staff to do, or organise, something for you and your peers; for example, career fairs
- continually appraise your career choices objectively.

Components of career decisions

You may think that deciding on the career for you is all about choosing the specialty that you want to work in. If so, you are mistaken. Figure 3.1 illustrates multiple factors that you must consider when making career decisions. This is not exhaustive; there may be some factors that are not relevant to your interests or circumstances and many other factors that are not included, but will have a huge impact on which career is right for you. Try to refer back to this diagram when you are making career choices in the future to make sure you have evaluated the potential job as thoroughly as possible.

Information regarding careers, individual specialties and conditions can be found in journals. All university and hospital libraries should have a good selection of medical, medical career or related journals; if not they should be able to obtain any requested. In addition, electronic versions of many journals can be obtained through the National Library for Health (NLH) (www.library.nhs.uk).

The aim of the NLH is to provide clinicians, medical students, patients, carers and the general public with access to the best current know-how and knowledge to support healthcare-related decisions. It is also useful for healthcare professionals who are working in the private sector where common standards should apply. You should make time to investigate these resources as they may not only help with your studies, but also with your future career decisions and management.

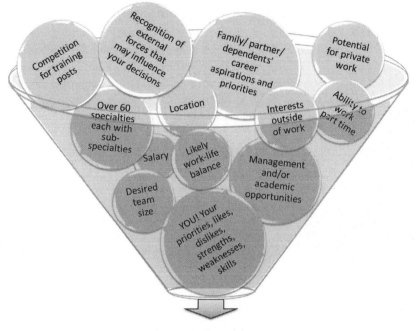

Career Decision

FIGURE 3.1 Factors to be considered when making career decisions

GATHERING CLINICAL KNOWLEDGE

An immense amount of information is out there. Information can be gained by reading journals regularly, which will keep you up to date with current practice; journals can often provide career ideas or points for thought. If you have a specific area of interest it is probably worth looking through a few relevant journals before handing over the cash for a subscription. Journals will provide you with insight into whether a particular specialty interests you.

Journals that medical students may find useful include:

- *British Medical Journal* (BMJ) (www.bmj.com/) – this contains news and research on any aspect of medicine, also contains a dedicated section for career articles as well as listings of jobs nationally and some international jobs
- *Casebook* (www.medicalprotection.org/uk/education-publications/casebook) – you will receive this for free if you are a member of the Medical Protection Society
- *The Foundation Years* (www.medicinepublishing.com/home/journals) – the content of this journal corresponds with components of the Foundation Programme syllabus

- *The Lancet* (www.thelancet.com/) – an independent medical journal detailing research and reviews
- Medicine Publishing has a range of journals targeted at specialty groups including medicine, surgery, psychiatry, anaesthesia and paediatrics (www.medicinepublishing.com/home/journals) – each journal has themed issues detailing up-to-date information on the management of conditions grouped by sub-specialty
- *Student BMJ* (http://student.bmj.com/) – covers all areas of medicine and surgery at a medical student level.

GETTING INTERACTIVE

Throughout this book you will be told that thinking about your future career cannot start early enough. You should learn to take a critical and reflective look at your motivation, skills and aptitudes to help assist your career progression. Not only that, but career development is an ongoing process that evolves and progresses with each learning experience. To help support your career development, reflection and contemplation, photocopy and complete the forms found in Appendices 2 and 3. For the most beneficial results, complete these in your own time and as honestly as possible.

We suggest that the 'Current career interests' form (*see* Appendix 2) is best completed at the following times:

- beginning of third year (first clinical year)
- end of third year (first clinical year)
- end of fourth year (second clinical year)
- end of fifth year (third clinical year)
- end of Foundation Year 1
- end of Foundation Year 2.

We also suggest you complete the 'Using clinical attachments to further career development decisions' form (*see* Appendix 3) after:

- each placement or rotation
- each student-selected component
- your elective.

Each form takes only a few minutes to complete and this will be time well spent. Simply reading the forms and providing answers will stimulate you to consider your current career development situation and assist with job applications in the future.

Reflection should form an important part of your progress through medical school and your future career. However, anecdotally, it often seems to be something that students think they can't do, don't want to do or that it is a waste of time. Reflection on positive, negative and challenging situations and subsequent development of learning needs and ways to address these are essential to being a life-long learner, improving your professionalism and directing your postgraduate training. If you have regularly done reflection as a student, you have a good evidence base on which to make clinical decisions. Reflection on yourself, your abilities and your likes and dislikes is the foundation to your career decisions. How do you know what you want to do or what you really don't want to do? The answer is: through reflection of previous experiences and skills that you know you do or do not possess.

Reflection holds the key to future job applications. Many application forms require you, for example, to discuss previous experiences and how this will make you a better doctor or how your experiences have led you to want to apply for that post. In Appendix 4 and Appendix 5 you will find two templates that you may wish to use in your reflective process. The former is for those of you who are less practised in the process of reflection. Once you feel more confident, try the form in Appendix 5.

HOW COMPETITIVE IS YOUR DESIRED SPECIALTY?

At present there are over 65 specialties, but how competitive is it out there?

This is a difficult question, not least because competition ratios are a dynamic entity. If a specialty is highly competitive one year, it is entirely possible that the following year the competition ratio may decrease significantly as applicants were 'scared off' by the previous year. In addition, workforce planning in the NHS results in variable quantities of specialists being required in each specialty; this alters the number of posts available and thus the competition ratios even when the number of applicants remains constant.

When using competition ratios, medical students and junior doctors should be warned not to use these as a sole decision-making tool. Many factors should be taken into consideration when choosing your future long-term specialty, including your ability and desire to undertake it, the location of training and the work-life balance that the specialty is likely to provide. Therefore, do not let the competition ratio – a value that can change tremendously year on year – be the decider of your destiny.

Competition ratios for unit of applications and specialties for Specialty Training Year 1 will be demonstrated here. The Modernising Medical Career (MMC) website (www.mmc.nhs.uk) gave encouraging information to Foundation doctors by saying that in 2008 most would get a job in Specialty Training. However, Foundation doctors were warned that to get a job they would have to be prepared to be flexible about where they did their training and in which specialty.

Figure 3.2 demonstrates the competition ratios for Specialty Training Year 1 for each unit of application in 2007, based on figures published by the MMC, which were accurate in March 2007. On average, there were 6.4 applications and 1.7 first choice applications for each post. London and Kent, Sussex and Surrey (combined) had the highest ratio (n=2.3) of first choice applications to posts and Trent and Eastern both had the lowest ratio (n=1) of first choice applications to posts. In total, 50% of first choice applications were shortlisted with a range of 38% (Oxford) to 69% (Leicester).[1]

Figure 3.3 demonstrates the competition ratios for Specialty Training Year 1 for each specialty in 2007, based on figures published by the MMC, which were accurate in March 2007. Public health had the highest ratio (n=5.4) of first choice applications to posts and surgery in general with the theme of trauma and orthopaedics had

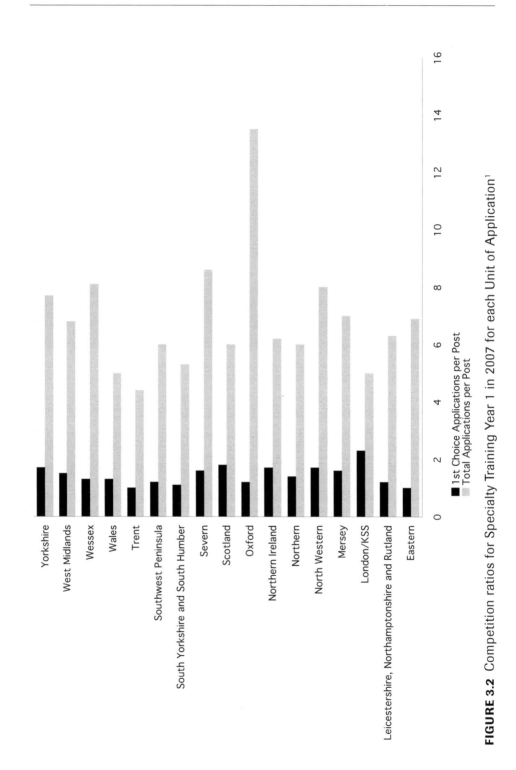

FIGURE 3.2 Competition ratios for Specialty Training Year 1 in 2007 for each Unit of Application[1]

the lowest ratio (n=0.6) of first choice applications to posts. In total, 50% of first choice applications were shortlisted with a range of 19% (public health and clinical radiology) to 74% (general practice).[1]

The British Medical Association's June 2008 report of the 2006 Medical Graduate Cohort Study describes the most popular long-term specialty choices of 403 responding Foundation Year 1 doctors as general practice (28%), general medicine (15.1%) and surgery (10%) as the most popular. The least popular choices were pathology (0.2%), geriatrics (0.7%) and public health (1.0).[2]

Specialty competition ratios may be found on the MMC website (www.mmc.nhs.uk) and/or on individual deanery websites. Further related information may also be produced by the British Medical Association (www.bma.org.uk).

MATCHING PERSONALITY TYPE TO CAREER

Analysing your personality may fill you with fear. You may be worried you will discover a hidden secret! Maybe you feel uncomfortable with the potential for being labelled and/or stereotyped. However, understanding your personality can benefit both you as a medic and your patients. Anita Houghton states that by understanding and evaluating your personal style and preferences you will quickly and more easily be able to understand and value others more. As a result you will have increased productivity, improved working relationships and a happier, more fulfilled working life.[3]

This section of the chapter will introduce a resource that you can use to identify and understand your personality type and/or likely specialty preferences. However, this section must also come with a warning. The exercises and resources introduced are not prescriptive; they will not tell you which career is best for you. They should be used to highlight possible avenues to pursue further and should be a trigger for you to think hard about your personality, strengths and weaknesses and how these fit in with different specialties. The output for all of these exercises is only as reliable as the information that you input. Try to think hard about the answers to questions asked of you and take the exercises seriously.

Sci59

The Open University has produced an interactive package that uses a form of psychometric testing. The Sci59, Specialty Choice Inventory, requires you to comment on 130 statements that have been designed to identify the job attributes you value most highly. These are then correlated to 12 dimensions, helping you to recognise specialties that may be your best (and worst) matches. The ensuing report that is automatically generated contains four sections:

1   Full listing – lists all specialties from 1–59 with 1 being the specialty you are most suited to as a result of your answers, and 59 being the specialty you are least suited to
2   Comparative – lists the top 10 specialties most suited to you with three traits that are required to work within this specialty
3   Results – lists the top and bottom 10 specialties most and least suited to you, respectively

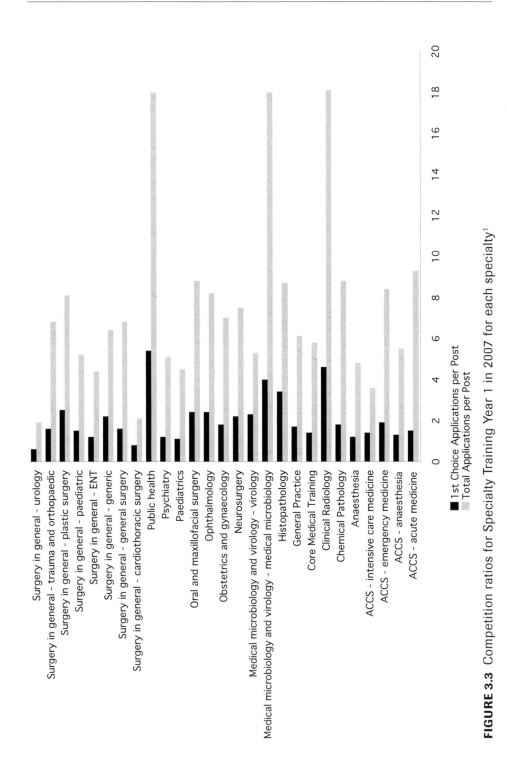

FIGURE 3.3 Competition ratios for Specialty Training Year 1 in 2007 for each specialty[1]

4   Graph – provides you with information on your strengths and weaknesses in each of the 12 dimensions, based on the answers given. A score of 50 is the average for the population, a score of less than 50 indicates this parameter may be a weakness for you; a score of more than 50 may indicate you have strength in this parameter.

The maximum benefit of Sci59 can only be gained if you not only look at the specialties suggested, but also reflect on why this is the result that your answers provided. A suggested method of interpreting the results of the Sci59 is:

1   Reflect on your strengths and weaknesses that are demonstrated by the graph. Do you think these are fair, accurate and/or true? If not, why do you think your attributes have been demonstrated incorrectly? Can you think of examples from your past experiences to refute the results given here? Have you been realistic about your best and worst attributes? Make sure you know your actual strengths and weakness and not just those that you desire. If you have a weakness that you wish you didn't, now that you have identified it you can do something to improve your skills in that area, if possible

2   Look at the specialties that are listed as your top 10. Are any of these surprises? If so, look at the comparative results to see which traits of yours correlated with those required for the surprise specialty. Can you see now why this specialty featured in your top 10?

3   Now try to identify why your bottom 10 results are listed as such. Again, are there any surprises? If yes, were any of the bottom ten specialties you were considering for your long-term career? If so, this should not necessarily make you change your mind, but you should definitely seek advice if you plan to continue pursuing this specialty as a career. There is such diversity within each specialty that even if your attributes appear to make you an unsuitable match, there may be a sub-specialty that is perfect for you

4   Finally, look at the full listing. Are your thoughts about the specialties that may be suited to you correlating well with where they rank? Have you had enough experience of the specialties ranking as being most suited to you to be able to know whether they are likely to be right for you? If not, have a think about arranging some time in that specialty.

If you like the sound of Sci59 the bad news is that it is password protected and passwords come at a cost. However, the good news is that some medical schools and deaneries, for example, West Midlands Workforce Deanery, have bought large numbers of passwords to allow students and junior doctors free access. If you are interested, try contacting someone at your deanery or medical school career department to see if a password is available for you. If not, the British Medical Association (BMA) has provided free access to its members through its career pages on-line (www.bma.org.uk). Each password allows you four uses over two years.

For more information about the Sci59 and details on how it was developed visit the website http://sci59.open.ac.uk.

The Myers-Briggs type indicator

The Myers-Briggs type indicator (MBTI) is a framework that describes four areas in which people differ (extroversion/introversion, sensing/intuition, thinking/feeling and judging/perceiving) and labels personality depending on these differences. The MBTI is a well-endorsed and frequently used psychometric test.[4] Your 'type' is merely a collection of approaches or practices that you prefer to carry out, which only you can identify. In reality, these preferred approaches co-exist so we express more than one personality type in different settings and circumstances. However, we usually display a single dominating preference for a particular 'type'. These preferred approaches are nothing to do with our abilities, which are a completely separate issue. It is important to realise that we can all be taught approaches or practices preferred by our opposing types.

So, what is your type? Anita Houghton published a fantastic series in the *Student BMJ* called 'Understanding Personality Type'. Her insightful work has been summarised in Table 3.1, Figure 3.4 and Figure 3.5.[3,5–10] Read the statements in Table 3.1, 'Personality toolkit', and tick only those that you honestly believe describe you. Then refer to Figure 3.4 and follow the flowchart based on the answers you ticked to find out what personality type you predominantly are. Figure 3.4 also highlights some of the traits that constitute that type: qualities that you may discover describe you accurately. Reflect on these traits; can you identify them within yourself? Had you realised you owned these traits before?

Once you have discovered your predominant personality type you can use this information constructively to assist you in maximising your efficiency and efficacy at work. Houghton identified a number of tasks and activities that take place every day in medicine, which are presented in Figure 3.5. Knowing which of these are preferred by your personality type allows you to consider the areas of medicine in which your strengths lie, and therefore, which future career may best suit you.

If you are interested, the full articles are well worth a read as they go on to explain how you can make the most of your personality traits as well as how to cope when undertaking tasks that are not suited to your personality. To discover even more about your personality type, all 16 type descriptions may be found on a website (www.capt. org/mbti-assessment/type-descriptions.htm).

What is the best personality type to be? For you, it is the type you really are. The most rewarding experiences you have will be those that come through the strengths that constitute your personality type.[11] Just remember that preferred approaches to thinking, acting and decision-making are not abilities. We can all be taught approaches or practices that are outside those we prefer when the situation demands.

Windmills online

Windmills online (www.windmillsonline.co.uk) is an interactive online resource that helps you to evaluate your current career position and the direction you should go from here. There are three main sections: Where am I? What sort of life do I want? How can I start working towards my kind of life? The resource contains main questions that should really get you thinking about basic career-related topics and it cannot help but trigger you to evaluate yourself and your current position along your career journey.

Many medical school and deanery staff are now being trained in the Windmills course so that they can deliver a similar approach in a more personal basis. Look out for sessions being held locally; they are well worth attending.

TABLE 3.1 Personality toolkit[3,5-10]

1a	I really enjoy teamwork and mixing with lots of people at work/university/socially
1b	I like days when I have the chance to read, reflect, study or write
1c	If a new person joins the firm/group I'm the first one to approach them, welcome them and invite them to tonight's social event
1d	On a ward round, when the firm is asked a question, I think through my answer carefully before speaking
1e	A day full of action and interacting with loads of people is draining
2a	I prefer lectures/talks to provide information in a detailed, stepwise and factual manner
2b	I am always full of new ideas, different ways of doing things and focus on tomorrow
2c	When given data I like to create patterns and meanings associated with it, and develop theories and possibilities
2d	I trust experience and tried and tested methods of doing things
2e	If someone were to ask me to describe an object I would give a precise description of what it looks like and its exact function
3a	I make decisions based on what is the most logical thing to do rather than how it will affect others involved
3b	People describe me as reasonable, fair and objective, and I like to be complimented for my competency
3c	I enjoy talking to patients and relatives
3d	People describe me as compassionate, tender and kind, and I like to be complimented for these qualities
3e	I am guided by values rather than cause and effect
4a	I like to have a clear plan of what I am doing and when; to have organisation and structure in my life
4b	I adapt to change easily; I am good in emergencies and filling in at the last minute
4c	I like being prepared and getting jobs done
4d	I feel constrained by schedules and like to keep my options open
4e	I am flexible, spontaneous, and feel energised by last-minute pressures

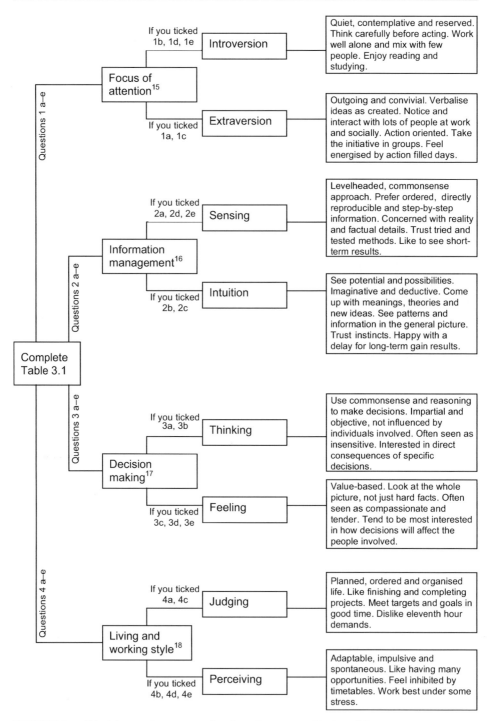

FIGURE 3.4 Working out your predominant personality type[5-8]

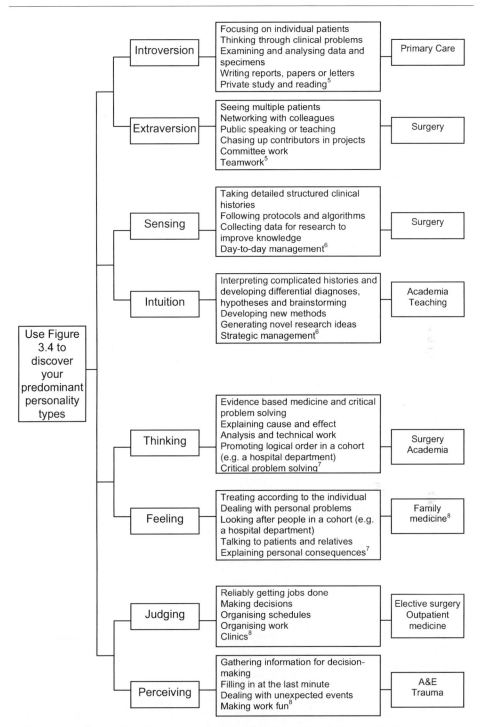

FIGURE 3.5 Examples of components and areas of medicine suited to particular personality types[5-9]

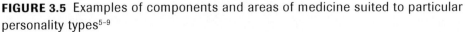

SORTIT

The University of London Careers Department present SORTIT (www.careers.lon.ac.uk/sortit), an interactive resource that has been designed to help you in your career journey. Free registration means that your results are stored for future review. To learn more about you, your values, your skills, your working style and your personality, use the resources in the 'self-knowledge section'.

REFERENCES

1 Modernising Medical Careers. *Posts, applications and shortlisting information by Unit of Application for Entry Level ST1 posts*. Available at: www.mmc.nhs.uk/default.aspx?page=348 (accessed 12 January 2009).
2 British Medical Association Health Policy and Economic Research Unit. *Cohort Study 2006 Medical Graduates*. June 2008. London: British Medical Association; 2008.
3 Houghton A. Understanding personality type: introduction. *StudentBMJ*. 2004; **12**: 366–7.
4 Bess TL and Harvey RJ. Bimodal score distributions and the Myers-Briggs type indicator: fact or artefact. *J Pers Asses*. 2002; **78**: 176–86.
5 Houghton A. Understanding personality type: extraversion and introversion. *StudentBMJ*. 2004; **12**: 410–11.
6 Houghton A. Understanding personality type: sensing and intuition. *StudentBMJ*. 2004; **12**: 456–7.
7 Houghton A. Understanding personality type: how do you make decisions? *StudentBMJ*. 2005; **13**: 20–1.
8 Stilwell NA, Wallick MM, Thal SE, *et al.* Myers-Briggs type and medical specialty choice: a new look at an old question. *Teach Learn Med*. 2000; **12**: 14–20.
9 Houghton A. Understanding personality type: how do you like to live your life? *StudentBMJ*. 2005; **13**: 62–3.
10 Houghton A. Understanding personality type: how it relates to job satisfaction. *StudentBMJ*. 2005; **13**: 108–9.
11 www.capt.org/mbti-assessment/best-type.htm

FURTHER READING

Chambers R, Mohanna K and Field S. *Opportunities and Options in Medical Careers*. Oxford: Radcliffe Medical Press; 2000.
Cross P. Spoilt for choice. *BMJ Careers*. 2008. Available at: http://careers.bmj.com/careers/advice/view-article.html?id=3084 (accessed 12 January 2009). (Lots of hints and tips about choosing a specialty.)
Hopson B and Scally M. *Build Your Own Rainbow: workbook for career and life management*. 2nd ed. London: Kogan Page; 2000.
Houghton A. *Know Yourself: the individual's guide to career development in healthcare*. Oxford: Radcliffe Publishing; 2005.
Kendell E. *The Myers-Briggs Type Indicator Manual: UK supplement*. Oxford: Oxford Psychologists Press; 1998.
MacKinnon DW. Personality and the realization of creative potential. *Am Psych*. 1965; **20**: 273–81.
Myers IB and McCaulley MH. *MBTI Manual: a guide to the development and use of the Myers-Briggs type indicator*. 3rd ed. Palo Alto, CA: Consulting Psychologists Press; 1998.
Research centre for the Myers-Briggs type index (www.capt.org).

Preparation for future jobs

4

This chapter provides general advice for you to use when you are preparing to apply for jobs at any stage of your career. Consider the advice given here in conjunction with Chapter 11.

RECORD OF PROFESSIONAL DEVELOPMENT

It is never too early to start preparing for future jobs. The earlier you start the better. One way of preparing for job applications is by using a record of professional development (ROPD). Official ROPD folders are handed out in some medical schools to students in their pre-clinical years. If this does not happen at your medical school, you can easily create your own by buying a large ring binder or box file and some dividers.

If your medical school is more technologically advanced you may have an electronic ROPD or portfolio system; the principle remains the same.

The purpose of a ROPD is to collate information about your skills, achievements and interests. It is a record of proof to support what you have been doing throughout your training and career to date. You can then either take the whole thing to future interviews or use it to create a personal summary.

Information contained within your ROPD should include:
- a regularly updated CV (*see below*)
- summary of exam, project and assessment results
- copies of written projects, reports and published papers
- regularly updated career aspirations, strengths and weaknesses, and current views on your professional development; you could use the forms in Appendices 2 and 3, designed for this purpose
- details of skills you have which are relevant to professional development.

Set aside some time on a regular basis – maybe each time you get exam results – to go through your ROPD and update each section. It is easy to forget about relevant information if you do not complete this until the end of your medical training. It does not take long to keep your ROPD up to date and it will be incredibly useful to you. Carry on the collation of this information in your postgraduate career. The key to a successful ROPD is that it is contemporary and accurate.

CURRICULUM VITAE

Your curriculum vitae (CV)[1-6] is incredibly important. Despite the current trend of scoring systems and structured application forms for postgraduate job applications, CVs are often a major part of the contact you make when applying for jobs. In addition, the number of applicants to postgraduate posts is increasing.[6] It is crucial that your CV is accurate, current and gives a fantastic first impression.

You can also use your CV as a means of recording your achievements, experiences and skills to date. It can be useful to have a 'master' CV into which you enter everything you do. Then, when you have to fill out structured application forms or provide potential employers with a CV, you can extract the relevant details as appropriate to create a tailored document in the future.

Although there is no standard format, presentation or type of CV that will impress everyone,[6] the presentation and content can influence the chances of a successful application.

The first tip is *do not lie*. You must be ready to be asked about every single thing you write in your CV. If you are audited and found to be lying you may risk your registration with the General Medical Council (GMC).

When writing your CV, an important and useful starting point is to follow any instructions present in the job advertisement. Although obvious, this is not always done and can be a way for recruiters to weed out the first set of CVs for rejection.[7]

Nowadays it is expected that your CV is word-processed and printed on good quality paper. The use of a laser printer to print your CV is recommended; however, if you do not have one it is not necessary to use a professional company to produce your CV. Before you send it off, just ensure that there are no smudges. Tabulation, especially of qualifications and personal details, allows quick and easy reference. CVs that lack clarity, have an unstructured layout and are not easy to read, do not impress the recruitment team; factors such as these may result in an immediate rejection of your application regardless of the content.[6]

You must include information such as training and experience in specific and/or relevant areas to the job you are applying for. Often experience gained within posts is assumed; highlight anything particularly special or outstanding about any aspect of your particular job.[6] For example, if you have worked in the country's leading liver unit with a highly renowned hepatologist, point this out, otherwise someone may assume you worked in the gastroenterology department in a small district general hospital.

In apparent contrast to the above, it is important that you do not just include information narrowly involved with the specialty to which you are applying. Try and think a bit more laterally and include details of your experience and skills in allied specialties. You may wish to include work within varying populations, highlighting your broad clinical experience. Conversely, if your previous experience has not been directly related to the job, you should clearly justify how it is relevant to the post you are applying for. Your application will not be dismissed if you can prove that previous unrelated positions are not due to a failure in your career progression or indecisiveness (*see* Box 4.1).

BOX 4.1 Suggested information for inclusion in your CV

Curriculum vitae

Personal details:
- Names (first name(s), surname)
- Your main or most recent qualification
- GMC registration number, valid training permit, experience in the UK
- Postal address
- Telephone (landline and/or mobile), e-mail and fax (where applicable)
- Date of birth, age

Career details:
- Education:
  - qualifications, prizes, relevant non-academic achievements – GCSE/A-levels (or equivalent) become irrelevant, university degrees and grades are essential; BMedSci is less relevant if obtained through an integrated medical degree unless it resulted in first-class honours or a publication
  - courses
  - dates
  - institution and location
- Work history – in reverse chronological order – and can include elective, research and relevant part-time jobs (e.g. healthcare assistant, GP note summariser):
  - date
  - position
  - current employer's name and location
  - duties, achievements and experience – think about the following areas: leadership; self-motivation and initiative; time management; teamwork; teaching; communicating with patients and professional colleagues. Other than in surgery or anaesthetics, listing specific procedures you have performed is unnecessary; if applying for surgery or anaesthetics you should ensure you have an up-to-date log book to refer to
- Published work – holds more weight if published in reputable journal, quality is greater than quantity
- Clinical audit and research – valued equally, often only count if resulting in publication
- Courses and conferences you have attended:
  - dates

- locations
- names
- Presentations you have given
- Career aspirations:
  - brief statement – it may not be definitive in junior doctor years
  - include how you think the job will help you to achieve these aspirations

Additional information and useful skills:
- Clinical
- Computer
- Languages
- Management – this is not necessary as a junior doctor; however, it is a bonus
- Administration

Personal specification:
- Interests
- Desirable criteria – aspects of professional or personal life you are proud of
- Leisure activities

Referees – usually you require two, it is polite to ask permission first:
- Names – one should be your current boss or tutor; well-known or distinguished names can be good, if possible
- Postal address
- Telephone, e-mail and fax (where applicable)

As a medical student looking ahead at this chapter you are in an advantageous position because you have the time to plan and adhere to the advice being given. You can also ensure you work hard at preventing gaps appearing in your career pathway. However, sometimes gaps are unavoidable, and may have already occurred for the junior doctors reading this. To prevent these gaps holding you back you must be able to justify them appropriately when applying for future jobs. Depending on the reason for the gaps, you may be able to relate the experiences you gained during that time, or the problems you were having, to you being a better applicant now.

Any work in progress may be included on your CV, but exercise caution: work in progress may be interpreted as your inability to finish anything, or something that will interfere with the performance of your next post. Present your work in progress to demonstrate that you are a hive of activity and have constantly got something on the go. If you can show that there is an exciting piece of work that has not reached its conclusion at the time of the CV application, you may be asked about it at the interview.

Try hard to think of appropriate and useful qualities and experience that you have, which other applicants may not have. These may include projects, part-time jobs or voluntary work. You should aim to demonstrate an appropriate level of knowledge and experience. However, it is important that you can prove you are a well-rounded and a potentially invaluable member of the team.

Box 4.1 illustrates the type of information recommended for inclusion in your CV. This is a full illustration, demonstrating many aspects you may like to include, but very few people, especially early on in their career, will be able to write something under every heading. If all headings can be filled, your CV will probably be too long. Pick out the most important and relevant points to match the job specifications. Number the pages for ease of reference at an interview. Bear in mind, this is a highly personal document, so add in anything else you think is relevant and feel free to personalise the design of your CV. If you are unsure about the inclusion of certain personal information, ask senior colleagues for advice. You may also require advice from a medico-legal company depending on what your query is.

A word of warning: do not let your artistic temperament take over so much that your CV loses its professionalism. Consultants and others involved in recruiting you may not see your new-found favourite font in bright pink as 'cool' or 'funky' but more as 'strange', 'juvenile' or 'pathetic'. However, some people may use colour or include a photo in order to make their CV stand out. You will have to critically consider the use of such things in each case.

Finally, before you send off your CV, check it for errors in spelling, grammar and formatting. Although useful, computer spelling and grammar-checking functions are not foolproof; for example, they do not pick up errors in spellings that have resulted in a wrong but recognised word. Use an A4 envelope to prevent excessive creases in the document. Your CV will be more striking if it is a crisp, crease-free sheet.

INTERVIEW SKILLS[7-10]

Interviews provoke a reaction that is closely related to fear and terror in most people. Therefore, let us start on a positive note: if your application has reached the stage that you have been called for interview you have already impressed your potential employers. You can be safe in the knowledge that the information they have received from you so far has satisfied the basic requirements for the job.

So why do they need to see you? The two main aims of the interview process are:

1 to confirm whether you have the required professional competencies
2 to find out whether they think you would be a good colleague; that is, they want to explore your personality and attitudes.

The most important things you can think about before an interview are preparation and personal presentation.

Preparation

Preparation is key. Ever heard the old adage 'Fail to prepare, prepare to fail'? Nowhere is this more relevant. Do not attempt to go to an interview without preparing first. Preparation for your interview requires just as much attention as the earlier stages of your application. Preparation and accumulation of relevant knowledge enables you to feel and appear more confident.

You have probably already submitted a fair amount of information either via an application form or your CV, or both. You should be able to explain, in detail, everything you have included in these documents. Take a copy so that you can refer the interviewers to the relevant sections in answer to questions – they may not have had time to read them in detail.

Areas in which it is a good idea to do prior research include the following.
- The actual job and your potential role in that job. You could:
  - contact people in the department
  - contact the person currently in the job you are applying for
  - find out about the bulk of the work in terms of conditions encountered and procedures performed
  - determine which proficiencies and skills are required for the job and, if you do not possess them, whether training for these occurs in the post
  - recent, relevant journals
  - 'hot topics' in the news, relevant to the job or specialty you are applying for
  - influential past and present research in the relevant specialty
  - broad knowledge of the health service, including current debates and forthcoming developments.
- Questions, especially obvious ones, are a common area in which lack of preparation presents a major stumbling block in an interview. Although you do not want to rehearse the answers word for word, prepare rough answers for the most predictable questions. Some of these, and some advice regarding the answers, may include:
  - 'Why do you want the job?' – just do not mention pay, no overtime, good-looking nurses, etc.
  - 'Why do you want to work in this hospital or practice?' – think about the experiences provided by the service that interest you
  - 'What qualities do you have which you could bring to the job?' – 'Someone to have a good night out with,' will not impress the interview panel, no matter how young they are
  - 'Where do you see yourself, career-wise, in the future/in 5 years/in 10 years?'
  - 'What are your biggest achievements?' – these can be career- or non-career related
  - 'How do you manage stress?' – the better applicants will not mention alcohol
  - 'What are research and audit? What are the differences between the two?'
  - 'What is clinical governance?' – this is a 'hot topic' and it is important you understand at least the basics of it

- 'How would you describe your personality?' – highlight traits useful to the job
- 'What are your strengths?' – use the forms in Appendices 2 and 3 to assist in your answers to this question and the next one
- 'What are your weaknesses?' – try not to use 'being a perfectionist', it is a common, boring and predictable answer to which an interviewer's equally boring and predictable response will be 'What is your second weakness?'
- 'Do you have any questions?' – do not ask too many, but areas you may consider are: the particular clinical or research interests of the consultant or department; opportunities to gain experience in areas of particular interest to you; the nature of senior on-call support; educational, study and training sessions provided.

- The format of the interview itself. Not only will this prepare you so you can avoid any shocks, but it will also allow you to try and anticipate potential questions even more accurately. Try to find out what the format of your forthcoming interview is and if possible speak to those who have previously undertaken the same interview format for details of the type of preparation required. Formats of interview can include:
  - Informal chat – you and one or two other people talking in a more informal environment. Do not be fooled that you can act informally. This may be a more relaxed environment than other interview styles, however, you are still being analysed for your suitability for a job
  - Large panel – you will be interviewed by around five people for the entire process. Sometimes one or two of the interviewers take the lead with all the questions; in other situations all interviewers will be given a different subject area to question you about. This can feel quite intimidating as it can feel as if they are ganging up on you; however, you must remain confident within reason. Try to address each one of the interviewers in turn while giving your answer
  - Multiple panel – this is akin to an objective structured clinical examination (OSCE), in which you will be given a few minutes in front of a number of small interview panels. Each panel will undertake questioning of a certain area or will be marking you as you demonstrate a particular skill. You may be required to do anything from critically describing a recent journal article you have read, right through to practical demonstration of a clinical skill.

Personal presentation

Advice on personal presentation for an interview encompasses behavioural and aesthetic aspects.

First impressions really do count. You do not want to be late, so leave plenty of time for your journey, getting lost and finding somewhere to park. Ensure that your mobile phone is switched off. When you enter the room, despite how you may be feeling, try to appear confident, with a warm smile. Offer a handshake when being introduced to each interviewer.

Be polite at all times. This includes not making any jokes that have the potential to offend anyone, even slightly. Ensure that you sit upright and that your posture (and answers) portrays openness and honesty. This may include not crossing your legs. Try not to fiddle with anything and keep your hand gestures contained and to a minimum. When answering questions ensure that you look around at the whole panel and try to gain good eye contact if your interviewers are willing to engage in this.

Consider your choice of outfit. Men should always wear a suit or smart jacket and trousers. A tie is essential, but comic ties have no place. Women should wear suits or at least a smart, matching jacket, but do not have to wear skirts. Smart trousers or dresses are acceptable. Neither gender should be wearing clothes with logos or slogans. Be comfortable with what you are wearing so you are not tempted to adjust items of clothing during the interview. Your overall look should be clean, tidy and well groomed. Avoid bright colours in your hair, polish your shoes and do a final check for hanging threads, laddered tights or labels hanging out the back of the garments you are wearing.

Don't forget your behaviour may be monitored at every stage of the interview process. Be polite during all correspondence you have regarding the interview both before and after the event. Your behaviour may be observed even while you are waiting in holding areas prior to and following the interview proper, so ensure you remain professional and considerate at all times.

HOW TO DEAL WITH REJECTION[11]

Unfortunately rejection is common during a career in medicine. It can occur in response to attempts at publication, ideas for development as well as after job applications. This situation is not set to change in the near future, as more applicants are being rejected due to increasing numbers of applications for posts in the UK.

Everybody deals with rejection differently. Common feelings following rejection include negative emotions, such as sadness, anger and frustration, reduced motivation and doubts about self and career, perhaps leading to affected performance in your current job. None of these responses are problematic unless you experience them for a prolonged period of time. However, if negativity persists it may lead to depression, financial problems and further career problems. Haq and Agell[11] suggest the following practical steps to assist you with dealing with rejection.

- Share your feelings – a problem shared is not always a problem halved; however, sharing your feelings with other people opens up the opportunity for them to give advice. They may have been in a similar situation or be able to provide you with a different perspective, which may help you view your situation more positively.
- Seek advice from your mentor (*see* Chapter 6) or senior colleagues.
- Remind yourself of your strengths; the 'Current career interests' form in Appendix 2 will help you. You may have been rejected on only minor points. As you are good at many things, you should concentrate on these skills and abilities at times when you are feeling low in self-esteem.
- Assess whether or not your negative emotions are leading to depression. Seek

help if you, or your friends or colleagues, are concerned.

● Prepare for financial problems in advance, decide upon a strategy in case of rejection before the application process begins.

Lastly, there are various support groups open to you. You may find a source of support internally through the trust you belong to or through external support groups, like the Doctors' Support Network. This provides an independent, friendly and supportive service run by volunteer doctors. (*See* Appendix 1 for contact details.)

INTERNATIONAL GRADUATES AND THE 'PLAB TEST'

The Professional and Linguistic Assessments Board (PLAB) test is a two-part examination, set for non-European Economic Area (non-EEA) international graduates, in order to register with the GMC and compete for jobs in the UK.[12–13] The PLAB is designed to assess whether non-EEA international graduates have reached the minimum standard required in order to practise medicine safely in the UK.[12] Not all international graduates are required to take the PLAB, for example EEA graduates do not. It is up to each individual doctor to check with the GMC whether exemptions apply to them (www.gmc-uk.org/doctors/plab/index.asp).[13]

You need more than successful PLAB results, if applicable, to register with the GMC. First, you must have an 'acceptable primary medical qualification'. Non-EEA international graduates must also demonstrate good English language skills (satisfactory scores on in the International English Language Testing System [IELTS]). Finally, graduates should have 12 months' postgraduate experience as a preregistration house officer/Foundation Year 1 (PRHO/F1). Those without PRHO/F1 experience can still take the PLAB, but would need to apply for an F1 job, for which the competition is exceedingly high.[12]

The PLAB test itself is divided into two parts. The first is a written paper containing 200 questions of two styles: extended matching questions (EMQs) and single best answer questions (SBAs). SBA questions usually comprise no more than 30% of the paper. Part 2 is an objective structured clinical examination (OSCE) consisting of 14 five-minute stations. Although you may attempt Part 1 as many times as you wish, you must pass it within two years of passing your IELTS, when applicable. You may only take Part 2 four times and must pass this within three years of passing Part 1. If you fail four times you will be required to retake IELTS, if previously applicable, and Part 1 and Part 2 of the PLAB. Limited registration, from the GMC, must be granted within three years of successful completion of Part 2.

Passing the PLAB test does not automatically result in a job. In fact, because competition for jobs in the UK is so high, statistics show it takes at least six months to secure a job after passing the PLAB and many doctors do not have a job one year after. When accounting for the fees (over £500 for both PLAB tests plus the language exam), travel, visas and living costs, taking the PLAB test becomes very expensive.[12] The pass mark is set so that only a certain proportion of candidates pass at any one sitting. However, because the places are not rationed, many more people may take the PLAB test than there are medical posts.[12]

Useful experience can be gained by doctors in the UK by working on a clinical attachment. This is an unpaid post in which you can shadow a doctor. You can use this time to experience a specialty you have previously had an interest in to clarify whether or not it is for you, or use the time to familiarise yourself with the NHS and hospital procedures (clinical and administrative).[12]

Delays in taking up a given post may occur even when international doctors have passed the PLAB test and been appointed. Hospital trusts may have to undertake checks with the criminal records bureau, and various health checks, before allowing overseas-graduate doctors to have access to their patients. They may also require additional insurance cover before a clinical attachment can be started, but this is up to individual hospitals to decide.

For more information on the PLAB test and the information provided here, please refer to www.gmc-uk.org. Here you will find further, up-to-date information on what is involved, procedures, and sample questions and scenarios to help you prepare for both parts of the examination.

REFERENCES

 1 Houghton A. Getting that job: deciding to apply. *StudentBMJ*. 2003; **11**: 376.
 2 McErin S. Writing a winning CV. *BMJ Career Focus*. 2004; **328**: 225.
 3 Medical Forum. *CV Headings to Consider*. Available at: www.medicalforum.com/cv-headings.htm (accessed 8 February 2009).
 4 Turya E. Growing your CV. *BMJ Career Focus*. 2004; **328**: 226.
 5 Craft N. Making the shortlist. *BMJ Careers*. 1996; **313**: 2.
 6 Ariyasena H, Tewari N and Livesley PJ. The search for the perfect curriculum vitae. *BMJ Career Focus*. 2005; **331**: 167–9.
 7 Houghton A. Getting that job: preparing for interview. *StudentBMJ*. 2003; **11**: 414–15.
 8 Sudlow M. How to be interviewed. *BMJ Careers*. 1996; **313**: 2.
 9 Jewkes F. The advice zone. *BMJ Career Focus*. 2005; **331**: 64.
10 Thompson MJ and Heneghan C. Asking questions at the end of an interview for a clinical job. *BMJ Career Focus*. 2005; **331**: 67.
11 Haq SF and Agell I. Dealing with rejection. *BMJ Career Focus*. 2005; **331**: 75.
12 General Medical Council. *Guidance for PLAB Test Candidates*, updated July 2005. Available from: www.gmc-uk/org/doctors/plab/#2 (accessed 8 February 2009).
13 McGinn K and Haivas I. PLAB: key to the kingdom. *StudentBMJ*. 2005; **13**: 468–71.

FURTHER READING

Agha R. *Making Sense of Your Medical Career: your strategic guide to success*. London: Hodder Arnold; 2005. (Appendix 2 of this book details some questions often asked at interview.)
British Medical Association. Overseas doctors: sink or swim. *BMJ Career Focus*. 2004. Available at www.support4doctors.org/organisation.asp?id=115.
Burnett S. Dressing the part. *BMJ Career Focus*. 2005; **331**: 67.
Houghton A. Getting that job: the final offensive. *StudentBMJ*. 2003; **11**: 458.
Irish B. General practice: the bigger picture. *BMJ Career Focus*. 2005; **331**: 74. (Information for those considering a career in general practice.)
Poole A. What not to do at an interview. *BMJ Career Focus*. 2005; **331**: 65–6.
A survey of PLAB pass doctors may be found at www.gmc-uk.org

Career support, advisers and fairs

5

There are many opportunities available for you to obtain help and further information on career decisions and options. This chapter is designed to highlight the resources available to you.

CAREER SUPPORT

Access to career advice for both undergraduate students and postgraduate doctors has been limited in the past. Historically, the lack of appropriate career guidance has been well documented.[1] Most doctors report that they have never received any career guidance or counselling.[2] In a survey of BMA members, consisting of doctors and medical students, 95% of respondents reported that they had unmet career guidance requirements.[3]

The document *Signposting Medical Careers for Doctors*[4] highlights the recent situation; few medical students and doctors have access to impartial career advice and counselling, and they make career decisions based on 'preconceptions rather than sound judgement'.[4] They are often not aware of what is actually available or where to go for advice. Traditionally, career advice has been sought in an informal, ad hoc manner.

In a survey of BMA members, which included an assessment of views on previous career advice, respondents reported the following sources of career advice as being useful:[3]

- more experienced peers
- senior doctors
- doctors who are family or friends
- peer group members
- *BMJ Career Focus* (now accessible at http://careers.bmj.com/careers/hospital-medical-healthcare-jobs/html)
- university career advice
- medical career fairs
- career lectures at medical school.

Both students and institutions should adopt a pro-active and educational approach to career advice and guidance,[3] which should be incorporated into the medical school and Foundation training curricula. This means that fundamental changes have been, and should continue to be, made to career advice and guidance to make sure it is consistent, structured and clear as to who provides what. Some useful career advice is illustrated in Figure 5.1.

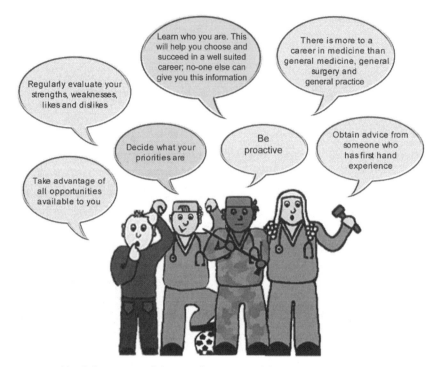

FIGURE 5.1 Useful career advice and opportunities

As a result of the *Modernising Medical Careers* (MMC) initiative, there has been a great move towards improving the level and standard of career advice made available to medical students and doctors at all levels of training. The provision of career advice is an integral part of the new medical career structure and, hence (thankfully) career support continues to be important as an expanding issue. Changes occurring as a result of this include the allocation of funding for a career adviser in each deanery.

Career Management: An Approach for Medical Schools, Deaneries, Royal Colleges and Trusts,[5] produced by the MMC Working Group for Career Management, highlights and suggests potential approaches to the delivery of career management initiatives for doctors between August 2005 and the end of 2007.[6] MMC guidelines (June 2005)[5] state that medical schools should be responsible for the delivery of career guidance by providing information and support to students in the following key areas:

- implementing career management initiatives by integrating them into the medical school curriculum
- developing the knowledge and skills required during undergraduate and postgraduate training
- developing the skills required by those giving, or likely to give, career information, advice or guidance
- encouraging students and developing their awareness and insight of personal strengths and weaknesses (*see* the 'Current career interests' form in Appendix 2

and the 'Using clinical attachments to further career development decisions' form in Appendix 3) and how these correspond to the variety of career opportunities there are in medicine.

With regard to postgraduate deaneries: these have a responsibility, along with medical schools, to provide support for medical graduates' transition into employment in their Foundation Training Course. You should expect:[6]

- focused postgraduate curricula activities, including those that broaden your understanding of postgraduate medical education and what it means in practical terms for you
- active facilitation and support of career management, with an impartial perspective and advice to signpost and support career networks (online, peer group, one-to-one career activities) which can help progress the continuing career interests and professional aspirations of doctors
- access to relevant and accurate sources of information when making a choice of medical career.

These processes are not mutually exclusive. In fact, they form part of the career development continuum. The division of responsibility at different phases in training means that career progression is not always addressed adequately.[3] Good communication, a good framework and commitment to career support is needed by both undergraduate courses and postgraduate deaneries to provide integrated services and prevent fragmentation of advice and guidance.

There has been more of a support structure for Foundation doctors rather than undergraduate medical students, but the resetting of this imbalance is continually being addressed.

What you should expect

According to *Career Management: An Approach for Medical Schools, Deaneries, Royal Colleges and Trusts*, produced by the MMC Working Group for Career Management,[5] there is a delivery model consisting of 14 components that should provide individuals with all the information, support and confidence needed to make informed and successful career choices. These include the following.

- Career information sources: these should cover job availability and training requirements and qualifications needed for different specialties, competition ratios and personal perspectives of posts (*see* boxed specialty profiles) as well as career pathways.
- Career conferences: events designed for undergraduate medical students and Foundation doctors to learn about different specialties, be involved in workshops (CV, interview, management skills) and debates.
- Career forums: provided as a rolling programme of events covering the main specialties. A career forum is a source of career information and a resource that encourages exploration of career options for senior undergraduates and Foundation doctors.

- Career handbooks: these should cover all the aspects of a career in medicine that are found in this one!
- Online guidance and career discussions: a range of adequately prepared individuals can be contacted to provide information and discuss career topics of interest nationally.
- Peer group activities: for both medical students and Foundation trainees. These provide a supportive career management environment where career exploration, development of skills and, later, discussions on career decisions can take place.
- Specialist career planning tools or programmes: help to develop good career decisions through the use of tools such as the personality toolkit, the 'Current career interests' form, the 'Using clinical attachments to further career development decisions' form and the Sci59.
- Focused experiences: *see* Chapter 10.
- Designated career advisers: see below.
- Designated trained career contacts: more targeted one-to-one advice in the form of clinical staff and non-medical professionals – *see below*.
- Medical school support services: integration of career management will be facilitated by student support and guidance through undergraduate, BMA, educational and academic committees and groups, as well as through occupational health, faculty and other pastoral support and guidance.
- Postgraduate deanery guidance and support services: support should be provided for trainees in difficulty through the use of career counselling, career tools and career development advice and facilitating access to a coach or mentor (*see* Chapter 6) and to occupational health services or a psychologist when needed.
- Occupational health and occupational psychology services: these are a source of external professional advice, especially when a doctor is unable to pursue a specific career option due to physical or mental health problems.

Via the MMC initiative, a mechanism is in place to co-ordinate career advice efforts on a national level. The aim is to abolish the current situation, in which there is a huge variety in the services provided by different deaneries. As a result, it is hoped that experiences will be shared and development costs reduced.

There are a large number of individuals who can provide career advice, information and guidance to medical professionals. Commonly, such individuals are clinical tutors of particular specialties. Key career support organisations also have at least a minimum level of career guidance skills and are aware of best practice in the giving of career information and advice. These are noted in *Career Management: An Approach for Medical Schools, Deaneries, Royal Colleges and Trusts*[5] and include the following.

- Your postgraduate deanery, including your Foundation Programme director, dean and associate dean: these may provide career information, career conferences, a career handbook, online guidance, peer group activities, specialist career planning tools or programmes, focused experiences, career advisers and designated trained career contacts, postgraduate deanery guidance and support services, occupational health and occupational psychology.

- Your medical school including any university career service that may be in place: these are able to co-ordinate career information, career forums, career conference, career handbook, peer group activities, specialist career planning tools or programmes, focused experiences, career advisers and designated trained career contacts and medical school support services.
- Medical royal colleges, faculties and institutions.
- Individuals, such as clinical tutors, educational supervisors (*see* Chapter 6), mentors (*see* Chapter 6) and career advisers.
- Career fairs.
- Student-selected components, electives, 'tasters', intercalated degrees, summer jobs, part-time work, work experience (*see* Chapter 10).
- NHS Careers: a good career information source which operates through a national call centre, website and free literature.[7]
- *BMJ Careers*.
- Medical Forum: an independent web service offering help with career planning, management courses, reviews and counselling.[8]
- The Association for Graduate Careers Advisory Services (AGCAS).
- The Institute for Career Guidance (ICG).
- The NHS trust employing you: they should provide career information, occupational health and occupational psychology services when it is appropriate.

Although the above list is a good starting point, to identify the appropriate organisations or individuals to assist you with career decisions, you should also look on notice boards, websites and in locally produced booklets for information on where further career advice can be sought.

What you can do

Although medical schools and deaneries have some responsibility to provide adequate career support for you during your training, this does not mean you can sit back and wait for help to come to you when you need it. You can help yourself and your peers through local activities. Examples of local career-related activities you may wish to get involved in include the following.

- Medical student career committee. For example, students at Keele University School of Medicine set up the Keele Medical Student Career Committee in March 2007. Through this committee students have raised questions and uncertainties they have about future careers and career pathways, set up their own career website (www.keelemedicalcareers.co.uk) containing useful career information, organised local career fairs, fed back ideas to influence the development of career support from the medical school and have been involved in the design stage of career research.
- Surgical society. All medical schools appear to have active surgical societies.

They are great for all students to become involved in as they often offer not only extracurricular surgical teaching, training and experiences, but also because they commonly have an active social calendar. If you are interested in being a surgeon, then being a member of the surgical society (or ideally part of the committee) is a very good idea.

- Medical society. For students interested in medical specialties there appear to be fewer active groups. However, this does not prevent you setting up your own medical society. You may wish to get together with like-minded students to organise extracurricular experiences in all medical specialties or one particularly specialty you may be interested in. Activities and experiences that you may find valuable to organise could include lectures from eminent clinicians, student case presentation sessions and practical skill workshops.

CAREER ADVISERS

Funding is given to deaneries for career management. One way in which they may provide this is to appoint specific career advisers. According to *Career Management: An Approach for Medical Schools, Deaneries, Royal Colleges and Trusts*,[5] the idea behind the career adviser's role is to:

- provide generic career advice to individual doctors
- respond to the initial career needs of medical undergraduates
- act as a signposting forum and referral point for more complex career-related requirements, such as human resources support
- address situations where no current career advice is being provided
- assist in career exploration through accurate information provision, encouraging reflective career progression and workforce profiling
- use career education and planning tools effectively
- promote consistent practice in screening individuals' readiness to make career decisions.

Career advisers are a useful source of advice and information as they are competent in a range of career management techniques and are aware of accepted good practice.

Designated trained career contacts provide more targeted one-to-one advice. They can give more skilled advice in placement issues, answer specific career queries, such as specialty advice, and provide targeted training co-ordination for those experiencing particular difficulties. They may also be able to provide confidential in-depth career counselling. In addition, some advisers may be trained in psychometric testing.

The MMC documentation[5] suggests that those who can deliver this service include the following.

- Appropriately qualified clinicians: these may include mentors, educational and clinical supervisors (*see* Chapter 6), clinical tutors, Royal College tutors and advisers, and associate postgraduate deans with specialty career interests.
- Clinical staff: nursing and allied health professionals who have worked closely with medical students and doctors.

- Non-medical professionals: qualified career advisers, experienced facilitators, HR representatives, postgraduate education centre managers and clinical education staff.

The amount of training designated career contacts receive depends on the institute. For example, trainee advisers at the University of Oxford attend a half-day course, whereas the University of Nottingham runs a series of courses covering counselling, career advice, how to access counselling and guidance facilities and stress management. The West Midlands Deanery provides formal training in advice and guidance for all associate deans and is interested in defining competencies for those giving career support.[3]

If you have not yet narrowed down your career choices, you may need to consult several advisers, or an adviser with a broader knowledge of a range of specialties.

Previously, there were serious concerns about the advice given by career advisers. These concerns are easy to understand as there was no regular monitoring of the quality of the advice given, nor any effective channel for trainees to voice their concerns.[9] With an explicit framework now in place and at least minimal training for anyone supplying simple factual career advice, as well as more thorough training for those providing in-depth career planning and counselling services, the situation should improve. However, not all consultants that you discuss career matters with, especially if in an ad hoc fashion, are skilled in appraisal or career counselling[10] and they may provide a biased view and judgemental opinion.[11]

You must learn to evaluate the information anyone gives you. It is also worth noting here, that in a study of the career intentions of pre-registration house officers (PRHOs; now known as Foundation Year 1, F1), the use of web-based career advice and Sci45, the predecessor to Sci59 (*see* Chapter 3) were more valued than career advice sessions. In fact, from 89 PRHOs who met either their clinical tutor or another career adviser, 83% found this source of career information or advice the least useful.[12] It is hoped that this view will change with the new reforms.

CAREER FAIRS AND EVENTS
Local

Educational supervisors, career advisers, undergraduate and postgraduate career leads and tutors should be advertising career fairs, forums and lectures at your university and/or hospital. If you are unaware of events held by your medical school or deanery first ask for information on organised events. If little has been organised or if what has been organised has not met your needs, you should request events that you believe would be helpful. You should never be worried about asking your medical school or deanery for help with your career development. You can make sure it is providing you with adequate career support, as detailed by the previous section in this chapter. If you want to supplement the activities of your medical school and/or deanery, consider setting up/joining a local career committee to organise events and resources as detailed previously.

Medical student societies, for example, surgical societies (known in some medical schools as 'SCRUBS' or 'SCALPEL') may organise career fairs. However, you must either ensure that they are not biased or, if you think they are, take any directed information with a pinch of salt.

The East Midlands Deanery offers an excellent example of how local careers services should exist and be delivered. They have a fantastically useful website, containing their own electronic local career handbook as well as details of local events. For example, they have a rolling programme, supported by the Medical Protection Society (MPS) and Medical Defence Union (MDU), which contains evening events that allow medical students and Foundation doctors to gain an insight into main medical specialties and specific career-related topics. It is strongly recommended that you visit the *Career Support* pages of the East Midlands Deanery website for further information (www.eastmidlandsdeanery.nhs.uk). In addition to attending such events, you should ensure that advice on CV writing and interview skills are provided too.

One successful way in which CV help and advice has been delivered was by the Keele Medical Student Career Committee (KMSCC). KMSCC organise a limited number of 1:1 slots during the career fairs that they host to enable students and junior doctors to take their CVs to professionals with knowledge of job application processes to gain feedback. The advice given is supplemented by a written handout that students and trainees can take away with them. This format of CV advice has been successful not just in the eyes of the trainees, but also the professionals providing the advice. Being local clinicians and/or faculty/deanery staff, the professionals enjoyed the opportunity to get to know local trainees better and to find out about their achievements, some of which are incredible and not previously known about.

Get involved: how to organise a career event

If you want to organise a career event the preparation must be arranged and targeted to the user group to make sure the event is a success. If you are going to organise a large event, such as a career event, you are definitely going to need help. Ideally you should form, or use, a pre-existing group or committee consisting of members of the target population, an administrative member of deanery or faculty staff and a clinician. This mix will ensure that the user group needs are met; you have easy access to medical school or local facilities; and your plans are realistic. To help get you started, below is a checklist of items that must be considered when planning a large career event, such as a local career fair.

- At least two to three months in advance: decide the target audience and the format of event (e.g. parallel sessions, lectures, sign-up sessions, stands); arrange a venue and book rooms thinking about the space required for the number of attendees you expect and to accommodate the format of your arrangement; decide on the topics to cover; invite organisations and clinicians requesting – where appropriate – funding and/or raffle prizes and/or pens to give out on the day; and get quotes for catering.
- One month in advance: advertise the events in multiple formats (e.g. posters, fliers, website, local newsletters, speak in lectures); consider asking delegates

to register to get an idea on numbers (not always reliable); ensure there is adequate car parking (try to arrange this to be free if possible); organise signposting to the event; confirm organisations' and clinicians' attendance and chase any funding that has been promised; gather material to create an accompanying book or pack and ask any presenters for electronic copies of their presentations; create forms/tickets/slips for the day (e.g. time slips, sign-up sessions, raffle tickets, suggestion/feedback forms); and book the catering.

- One week in advance: ensure availability of tables, chairs, boards, rooms and vacuum cleaner as required; buy incentives for evaluation sheet returns (e.g. lollies work well!); plastic cups, biscuits, bin bags, kitchen roll and cleaning wipes as required; and make a list of all the resources, paperwork and items you need to take with you.

- On the day: arrive at least one hour before the opening time of the event to ensure everything is set up when the first people arrive, photograph rooms digitally prior to moving furniture around to assist correct replacement; and delegate jobs to committee/group members to ensure all delegates, presenters and stand holders are greeted and know where to go and to undertake housekeeping duties (e.g. unwrapping food, tidying up); and to encourage sessions to run to time.

Regional

BMJ Careers has hosted regional career fairs in addition to its annual national fair (*see* next section). For example, the first West Midlands BMJ Careers Fair was hosted in Birmingham in October 2008. It is well worth attending regional BMJ Careers fairs as they offer a really comprehensive programme of seminars and courses with the benefit of limited travel to the event. Another benefit is that entrance to seminars may be subsidised for local doctors, whereas doctors from other parts of the country may have to pay. Find more information on planned events, costs, programmes and registration details for regional career fairs on the BMJ Careers Fair website (http:// careersfair.bmj.com).

National

Every autumn/winter BMJ Careers holds a national career fair at the Business Design Centre, Islington, London. This the largest medical recruitment fair in the UK. It runs a huge variety of seminars and hosts an exhibition containing multiple stands, thus providing such a vast range of career information that any career need will be satisfied, from choosing a specialty to improving generic skills (e.g. public speaking). Attendance to the exhibition is free if you pre-register for the day; however, delegates are asked to pay a small fee for turning up un-registered on the day and for attending the seminars/courses at the Career Fair. Information on charges is found on the website (http://careersfair.bmj.com).

BMA members can take advantage of the specialist careers information support available through BMA Careers Services. In addition to coaching and career tools, workshops are available (for a fee) to attend to improve your career related skills. A series of the workshops is targeted directly at junior doctors. For more information visit the BMA website (www.bma.org.uk/careers/careers_service/Careersworkshops.jsp).

The Royal Society of Medicine (RSM) runs a programme of events, including specific career meetings. These range from events that provide information on one or multiple specialties to events that cover specific topics, such as application advice. A full programme of events and details of costs (if any) of attending these sessions can be found on the RSM website (www.rsm.ac.uk).

Even for those of you who do not want to follow a traditional medical path or want to leave medicine, there is a national career fair that may suit your requirements. The *Alternative Career Paths for Doctors* career fair is hosted by Medical Success and provides information and advice about the options available to you. Delegates are required to pay to attend. For more information see the Medical Success website (www.medicalsuccess.net).

Do not forget that finding sufficient information about different specialties is worth little if you do not know enough about yourself. You have to be able to match your talents and abilities with the options available, both clinical and non-clinical. Now that you know what career support and information you should be getting, and where you can go to find it, the rest is up to you.

REFERENCES

1 Carnall D. Career guidance for doctors. *BMJ*. 1997; **315**: 6.
2 Allen I. *Doctors and Their Careers*. London: Policies Studies Institute; 1998.
3 Jackson C, Ball JE, Hirsh W, *et al. Informing Choices: the need for career advice in medical training*. Cambridge: National Institute for Careers Education and Counselling; 2001.
4 BMA Board of Medical Education. *Signposting Medical Careers for Doctors*. London: BMA; 2003.
5 Modernising Medical Careers Working Group for Career Management. *Career Management: an approach for medical schools, deaneries, royal colleges and trusts*. London: Department of Health; 2005.
6 www.mmc.nhs.uk/pdf/Career-Management.pdf
7 www.nhscareers.nhs.uk
8 www.medicalforum.com
9 Leung W-C and Birks K. Giving and seeking career guidance. *BMJ Career Focus*. 2001; **322**: 2.
10 Porter RW and Clayton B. Letters: career guidance for doctors. *BMJ*. 1998; **316**: 75.
11 Hutton-Taylor S. Do it yourself career guidance. *BMJ Career Focus*. 1996; **313**: 2.
12 Stern C. Career intentions of pre-registration house officers and the influence of career advice. *Br J Hosp Med*. 2005; **66**: 477–9.

FURTHER READING

Bache J. Choosing a career. *BMJ Career Focus*. 1999; **318**: 2.
Gale R and Grant J. *Sci45. The Specialty Choice Inventory: computer-based careers advice for doctors in training*. Milton Keynes: Open University Centre for Education in Medicine; 2001.
Turya E. *Your Career after PLAB: surviving tools for young doctors*. Manchester: Edukon; 2003.

Mentors and educational supervisors

Mentors can be an invaluable source of support during medical school. Later in your career, as a Foundation doctor, you will also receive support from an educational supervisor. This chapter sets out the factors that comprise a 'perfect mentor', how to find a mentor and why mentors are useful.

The BMA strongly advocates mentoring at all stages of medical education and throughout a doctor's career. In 2003, the BMA lobbied for the development of a mentoring system for all doctors and called on the government to resource it appropriately.[1] With increasing pressures on everyone's time, and the need to make career decisions earlier than before, mentoring provides both personal and professional support allowing individuals to develop knowledge, skills, attributes and enhance their practice.[2]

WHAT MENTORING IS

Mentoring has many definitions. The Department of Health (DoH) and the NHS value mentoring, and after an inquiry, the Standing Committee on Postgraduate Medical Education (SCOPME) defined mentoring as a:

> '... process whereby an experienced, highly regarded empathetic person (the mentor), guides another individual (the mentee) in the development and re-examination of their own ideas, learning, and personal and professional development. The mentor, who often, but not necessarily, works in the same organisation or field as the mentee, achieves this by listening and talking in confidence to the mentee.'[3]

In the most recent Modernising Medical Careers (MMC) publication, mentoring is defined as:

> '... a relationship where one individual (the mentor) guides another to explore and expand on their own ideas, so that they learn and develop both personally and professionally.'[4]

The list of definitions in both healthcare and organisation settings is extensive and they all sound rather similar. Collating the many and different explanations, the main elements which comprise mentoring include the following.[1,2,4–7]

● A professional relationship that should last over a fixed timescale, on a continuing basis and long term.

- Professional development, career progression and personal support:
  - mentoring should be a significant feature of an individual's career; especially at times of development, transitions and changes, for example between grades or placements
  - mentoring should help you to: take control of your career; understand how career choices are made and the wider socio-economic factors that may influence these choices; develop self-awareness and knowledge about your skills and abilities; investigate career pathways and opportunities and promote life-long learning throughout the career continuum
  - it should provide support to enable you to manage your own career by helping you develop effective career, life-planning and decision-making skills; this should occur through self-direction, personal control and responsibility.
- An opportunity to learn and develop whether your starting point is unsatisfactory or excellent.
- A mentor is generally a senior, experienced and respected member of the medical profession who can use their own experiences to guide the mentee to discuss, explore, develop, expand and later re-examine their own ideas and come to their own decisions. The mentee should not simply be told what to do.
- Issues should be explored in a constructive and non-threatening way.
- Mentor–mentee interaction should be confidential, so that the mentee can speak freely without fear of reprisal. Thus it should also be neutral and unbiased.
- Mentors and mentees should meet regularly, but not necessarily frequently.
- A mentor should be empathetic and someone who listens.
- Mentors and mentees need not be in the same organisation (and not in a direct management role with one another).

EDUCATIONAL SUPERVISORS

Educational supervisors are assigned to Foundation doctors, not medical students, and are concerned with helping you identify and meet your educational or training needs through a personal development plan.[5] The career support they provide is vital as they aid both career management and career education.

- *Career management* is a pro-active process entwined with career development. Your educational supervisor should guide you in how to manage your own career by helping you develop effective career, life-planning and decision-making skills through self-direction, personal control and responsibility throughout your career.[4]
- *Career education* occurs when educational supervisors help you to take control of your career by helping you to understand how career choices are made. This involves helping you to appreciate the wider socio-economic factors that may influence these choices, develop self-awareness and knowledge about your skills and abilities, investigate career pathways and opportunities, and promote life-long learning throughout your career.[4]

Some educational supervisors also provide career counselling and will assist you in reflecting on and evaluating your career and life plans, especially at transitions in your life. Others may give practical or emotional support, but this is not really in their remit. If you cannot find a mentor who covers the whole scope of mentoring, but are assigned an educational supervisor, make use of them. Regular appraisal is a good way to boost your morale and your motivation, providing that you are performing well.

In the following sections the term 'mentor' is used to cover all mentoring roles. Therefore, when career development is discussed, this term also includes educational supervisors.

WHY YOU SHOULD HAVE A MENTOR[2]

Everyone tends to be stressed these days. You may have too much to do and not enough time. You may not feel able to tell colleagues or medical friends how you feel for fear of being seen as weak. However, things can be different. The mentoring relationship provides you with the opportunity to share these feelings in confidence with someone who has dealt with them before. It gives you the chance to explore your real thoughts, express your views, test out ideas and raise questions you may not have previously considered. A mentor will give you the opportunity to reflect, allowing you to work through your own issues using a combination of support and challenges without them attempting to solve the problems for you. In this supportive and confidential environment you can take a step back and look at yourself honestly in all the roles that you perform. You may have serious questions about where you are in your career, where you want to go next and how to get there.

Mentoring is a professional support mechanism. It provides you with a port of call if you are encountering any communication or relationship difficulties, are having difficulties coping with stress, need help to avoid using adverse coping strategies (such as drink or drugs) or if you believe you are facing burn-out.

Finally, mentoring is a dynamic process; with each mentor–mentee relationship usually lasting about a year. Individuals' requirements change throughout their career; therefore mentoring can provide relevant and applicable guidance, ideas and advice at these junctures. This may also mean that at these different points in your career, you may need different mentors.

Mentoring is an essential component of career advice for both medical students and doctors. It has been identified as beneficial and advantageous as there is evidence of its positive effect in medicine.[6] The benefits of mentoring will invariably differ between individuals and different schemes. Such benefits are also difficult to quantify.

The possible benefits most associated with mentoring are:[1,2,4,7,8]

- Workplace benefit (e.g. improved work performance, relationships and communication)
- Acquisition of new or improvement of existing skills (e.g. encourages reflective practice and develops career planning skills)
- Improved learning opportunities (e.g. identification of specific educational needs)

- Career benefits (e.g. provides in-depth focus and support when making career decisions)
- Benefits associated with self-discovery (e.g. gaining a clear understanding of yourself)

Mentoring can be utilised to help support and promote cultural diversity or address issues of discrimination. Female consultants can provide mentoring to female junior doctors. Mentors from the same minority group as mentees can act as role models.

Traditionally, doctors have shown reluctance towards taking up mentoring schemes. Although this may be due to time constraints, it has been suggested that actively engaging in mentoring is seen as a weakness.[9] The potential advantages of mentoring need to be highlighted, with a wider range of information offered, in terms of the potential benefits and limitations of participation, so more medical students and doctors are willing to participate. 'Mentoring should be promoted as a positive and active method to enhance one's career.'[1]

FINDING A MENTOR

There is a vast difference in the way mentoring schemes are run between the various postgraduate deaneries.[1] In some deaneries, mentoring is part of the remit assigned to trusts and is not centrally co-ordinated. Many ad hoc mentoring projects also exist. Most mentoring schemes co-ordinated by deaneries were often targeted at consultants, whereas other schemes focused on overseas and international doctors or refugee and asylum-seeking doctors. Other postgraduate deaneries offered peer-mentoring schemes, a counselling service or did not offer a scheme but were able to refer doctors to relevant schemes that were available. Other mentoring schemes can be found through medical schools, royal colleges or individual trusts or departments. More recently, schemes have been designed to encourage a similar developmental relationship between peers.

So what situation are you in?

- You are already in a mentoring scheme. If this is so, use this chapter to maximise that experience. Make a list of objectives, if you have not done so yet, and go through all the different ways a mentor can be utilised. You should also evaluate your mentor–mentee relationship to date to see if it is working for you (*see below*).
- You do not have a mentor assigned to you.[2] You really should start doing some research into mentoring schemes that may be open to you, as the benefits of having a mentor are far-reaching.

Does your university, hospital trust or library have a list of individuals who are willing to be mentors? If not, is there anyone you know who has been a mentor before, or could fulfil the mentoring criteria? What sort of person do you need (*see below*)? In a survey of BMA members, consisting of doctors and medical students, 54% of respondents said they would go to senior doctors for advice; 21% would go to lecturers, trainers or tutors; and 6% said they would go to people in supervisory roles.[10]

When you have a shortlist, go and meet the individuals. Find out if they would be willing, and able, to commit to a voluntary mentor–mentee relationship. They must have the time and be enthusiastic about taking on the role. If they do not know about mentoring, find out what they think it entails, and take this Handbook with you!

See if you are able to build a rapport with your chosen mentor. Not only should it be someone with whom you would work well, they should be able to challenge you and make you think from different perspectives.

Ask if they have any previous experience of being a mentor, or indeed a mentee. Ask them how it went, what they can offer and about the opportunities for both of you. At different points in your career you may need different mentors. Not only that, but you may opt to have different mentors at the same time. This may be the case if they have different qualities, personalities or experiences, and can thus support you in different ways or for different aspects of either your personal or working life, or in your career.

A mentor can be any suitably experienced medical, allied health or non-medical professional and does not need to be in a managerial role in the same organisation as you.

MAKING THE MOST OF A MENTOR[2]

Traditionally, a mentor is an older and wiser colleague who can use their knowledge, skills and experience to empower the mentee.

Someone who has been a mentor before would be ideal as they should be well aware of how the relationship works. A degree of research is needed before you will find the right mentor for you, but it will be worth it in the end.

Box 6.1 contains lists of both essential and desirable qualities to look for in a mentor, as described in *The Good Mentoring Toolkit for Healthcare.*[2]

BOX 6.1 Qualities to look for in a mentor

Essential qualities

Impartial	Respectful	Ethical
Good listener	Effective leader	Supportive
Skilled in feedback	Interested	Non-judgemental
Perceptive	Able to challenge	Self-aware
Trustworthy	Chemistry (intellectual and emotional compatibility)	

Desirable qualities

Knowledge	Technical expertise	Instructor
Authority	Adviser	Seniority
Inspiring	Knows the health service	Experience
Patient	Able to receive feedback	

Discuss the terms of your mentoring partnership before commencing the relationship. By setting clear aims and objectives both of you will know what is expected and what needs to be achieved. These will not be the same for every person, or throughout their career, as each individual will have diverse requirements that will vary at different points in their career. This initial understanding will allow for a more successful and fulfilling mentor–mentee relationship.

First, set objectives covering the main purpose and focus of your meetings. Think about what you want to achieve in these sessions. For example, if you want to focus on career development you may want to answer the following questions.

● What is my ideal job?
● How do I get there?
● Do my skills and attributes suit this discipline?
● Do I want to tackle work-related issues, political issues, leadership styles, networking opportunities?

You should discuss the questions you have with your mentor and then plan when and how you want to cover them. This is a personal development plan. Think about whether you want to leave a set amount of time each session to discuss new issues. Prepare thoroughly for each session in order to get the most out of it.

Brief your mentor with your career aims, achievements to date, perceived weaknesses and strengths, and the nature of any advice sought in this area. This allows the mentor to research into any relevant issues or refer you to a more appropriate person if need be.[10]

REFERENCES

1 British Medical Association. *Exploring Mentoring*. London: British Medical Association Board of Medical Education; 2004.
2 Bayley H, Chambers R and Donovan C. *The Good Mentoring Toolkit for Healthcare*. Oxford: Radcliffe Publishing; 2004.
3 Standing Committee on Postgraduate Medical and Dental Education. *Supporting Doctors and Dentists at Work: an enquiry into mentoring*. London: Standing Committee on Postgraduate Medical and Dental Education; 1998.
4 Modernising Medical Careers Working Group for Career Management. *Career Management: an approach for medical schools, deaneries, royal colleges and trusts*. London: Department of Health; 2005.
5 Chambers R. *Survival Skills for GPs*. Oxford: Radcliffe Publishing; 1999.
6 Connor MP, Bynoe AG, Redfern N, *et al.* Developing senior doctors as mentors: a form of continuing professional development. *Med Ed.* 2000; **34**: 745–53.
7 Incomes Data Services. *Personnel Policy and Practice: mentoring*. Surrey: Unwin Brothers/The Gresham Press; 2000.
8 Oxley J and Fleming B. *Mentoring for Doctors: signposts to current practice for career grade doctors*. London: Department of Health; 2004.
9 Snell J. Head to head. *Health Serv J.* 1999; **109**: 22–5.
10 Jackson C, Ball JE, Hirsh W, *et al. Informing Choices: the need for career advice in medical training*. Cambridge: National Institute for Careers Education and Counselling; 2001.

7

What is good about a career in medicine?

Life as a doctor can be difficult. Colleagues, peers and other professionals moan about their work, life, pay and patients. The aim of this chapter is to provide you with the reasons why it is worth continuing in the medical profession and the benefits of working in the NHS.

To realise why this is a great time to be working in the NHS you should first consider the main criticisms of working in it and why these criticisms are becoming less valid.

Most doctors who have left the NHS blamed the poor lifestyle and low pay as their main reasons for leaving. However, Chapter 13 illustrates how these complaints are being vigorously tackled. Junior doctors' pay is now protected by the 'New Deal',[1] which results in them being paid for the hours that they work. The more antisocial hours you work the greater the supplement to your pay. You could end up being paid an extra 80% of your basic wage. The introduction of the European Working Time Directive (EWTD)[2] has resulted in junior doctors' hours being protected. In simple terms, they can no longer be made to work exhaustingly long hours. In fact, by 2009, the maximum hours a junior doctor will be allowed to work per week will be 48, a lot less than the 90+ hours per week of old!

The introduction of flexible working now means that you can work part-time without the fear of losing out on training. Not only may you want to undertake flexible training for childcare reasons, but also some people choose the flexible training route to enable them to pursue other interests half of the time. There are structured flexible-training arrangements in all deaneries (*see* the relevant deanery website for further details regarding eligibility for flexible training and the application processes for this).

The NHS doctors' representative organisations and doctors themselves realise that doctors need lives outside medicine. They need time with their families and to maintain other pursuits. The aim of the 'Improving Working Lives' initiative[3] is to let doctors live balanced lives. It sets out a standard against which staff can measure their trust's management of human resources. NHS organisations must prove how they are trying to improve the working lives of their employees.

No one can guarantee that by becoming a doctor you will have a brilliant life. However, what you can be sure of is that you will work in an environment that thrives on teamwork and close relationships. You will be immersed in a culture that believes in working hard and playing hard. However, there will always be people there to support you if your work or play begins to affect your life negatively, for example the Royal Medical Benevolent Fund (RMBF).[4]

Because of changes resulting from the Modernising Medical Careers (MMC) initiative (*see* Chapter 8), the time taken to become a consultant or GP, and thus attain your ultimate career goal, is now relatively short. In addition, the MMC initiative has encouraged the organisation of career pathways of doctors. The improved career advice from sources, such as this Handbook, specialised medical career advisers and medical career fairs (*see* Chapter 5), means there will be less confusion for potential and current doctors working in the NHS.

Revisit the usually stated reasons why it is good to work as a doctor in the NHS. You must have thought of some reasons why you wanted to become a doctor before you applied to medical school. Was it the job satisfaction, working with people who need your help, the status, the idea of making a difference to people's lives, the diversity and interests of various career pathways you can take, the achievements you gain along the way, the ability to work anywhere in the world, or just the big pay packet? From this nowhere near exhaustive list, it is plain to see that there are plenty of reasons why it is desirable to be a doctor in the NHS. This perhaps explains why applications to medical schools are always likely to remain high.

HIGH QUALITY CARE FOR ALL – 'THE DARZI REVIEW'

High Quality Care for All[5] is a report on a review of the NHS led by Lord Darzi, undertaken in partnership with patients, frontline staff and the public. It coincided with the 60th anniversary of the NHS and highlighted both the areas in which the NHS is succeeding and the areas requiring reform. The recommendations it makes are for locally, rather than nationally, led changes. It is an upbeat document in which the benefits of working in the NHS are made clear, for example:[5]

- increased numbers of doctors and other healthcare professionals have resulted in larger teams
- formalised multidisciplinary team discussion and interaction
- ability to provide more prompt treatment as waiting list times have reduced
- improved operative techniques have resulted in shorter admissions and quicker recovery for patients.

Although the reforms suggested are not taken as being positive changes by all clinicians, the report does recommend changes that will modernise the NHS. The fact that modernisation is being considered can only be constructive as social and disease demographics and expectations are changing.[5] Many of the recommendations are suggested to encourage effective, safe, easily accessible and timely services to patients through changing service provision and assessment of service. The recommendations are also designed to empower patients in being involved in and directing healthcare reforms. Some of the changes these recommendations may result in are controversial and do not directly improve the working life of NHS employees. However, recommendations that directly result in staff benefits are also outlined, which include:[5]

- provision of easy access to information about high quality care, a 'NHS Evidence Service' – a single web-based portal providing authoritative clinical and non-clinical evidence and best practice

- strengthening the involvement of clinicians in decision making at every level of the NHS
- placing emphasis on NHS staff to lead and manage the organisations in which they work
- a clear focus on improving the quality of NHS education and training.

It is strongly recommended that you read the *High Quality Care for All* report[5] as it is spelling out, in part, the future ahead of you.

REFERENCES

1 www.dh.gov.uk/en/Managingyourorganisation/Humanresourcesandtraining/ModernisingPay/DH_4053873
2 Department of Health, National Assembly for Wales, NHS Confederation, *et al. Guidance on Working Patterns for Junior Doctors*, 2002. Available at: www.dh.gov.uk/prod_consum_dh/groups/dh_digitalassets/@dh/@en/documents/digitalasset/dh_4069967.pdf (accessed 13 January 2009).
3 Department of Health. *Improving Working Lives Standard*, 2000. Available at: www.dh.gov.uk/prod_consum_dh/groups/dh_digitalassets/@dh/@en/documents/digitalasset/dh_4074065.pdf (accessed 13 January 2009).
4 www.rmbf.org
5 Department of Health. *High Quality Care for All: NHS next stage review final report.* Norwich: The Stationery Office; 2008. Available at: www.dh.gov.uk/en/Publicationsandstatistics/Publications/PublicationsPolicyAndGuidance/DH_085825 (accessed 13 January 2009).

FURTHER READING

Gray C. Life, your career and the pursuit of happiness. *BMJ Career Focus.* 1997: **315**: 2.

8

Medical career pathways

Great changes have occurred and continue to occur in medical career pathways. Major changes started with the Modernising Medical Careers (MMC) initiative. Since then, there has been contention, review and controversial suggestions for further reform. At the time of print the future medical pathways have still not been set in stone. This chapter will introduce you to the background to the reforms, the current training pathways and areas that may change.

WHAT IS MODERNISING MEDICAL CAREERS?[1-4]

In February 2003, the four UK health departments published a policy statement on *Modernising Medical Careers*. The aim of the MMC initiative was to improve patient care by delivering a modernised career structure with focused goals and objectives. The structured and streamlined, yet flexible, approach to training was developed to allow trainees to complete training schemes in the shortest time period possible while maintaining their professional competence (Figure 8.1). The structure that the MMC initiative provided ensured that there was less opportunity for 'drifting' to occur within a career.

Currently, all UK graduates are required to undertake the two-year Foundation Programme (*see* Chapter 9), and after successful completion of the programme trainees may enter specialist or GP training programmes.

Specialty and GP training programmes are delivered through a range of organisations, supported and overseen by the postgraduate deans. The administrative bodies responsible for delivering the specialty or GP training programmes may be known as a specialty or GP training school. Once doctors enter either of these programmes they have the opportunity to gain a Certificate of Completion of Training (CCT), subject to satisfactory progress. The Postgraduate Medical Education and Training Board (PMETB) has agreed the curricula of the specialist and GP training programmes; it is against the appropriate curriculum that trainees are assessed.

The number of years doctors will spend in training will vary depending on which programme they have undertaken. Once a doctor has received a CCT they are then legally eligible for entry to the Specialist or GP register and can apply for an appropriate senior medical appointment; this may include GP Principal, other employed GP, consultant or other specialist role.

The MMC initiative was designed to ensure quality-assured training. Thus the presence of general competencies, including the ability to manage acutely ill patients, is established using various assessment methods. Doctors training in a Foundation

Programme have to demonstrate possession of the attitudes and behaviours required to be a good healthcare professional before advancing into a Specialty Training programme. These competencies include accessibility, recognising one's limits, understanding equal opportunities and taking proper responsibility. This focus on competencies also ensures that practitioners can work in all settings, such as primary care and the community, in addition to hospitals. The types of skills that are assessed as a result of the MMC are:

● communication and consultation skills – with patients, families and colleagues
● teamwork – in uni- and multi-professional settings
● establishment and maintenance of effective relationships with patients
● use of evidence and data
● time management
● information technology (IT) skills
● patient safety – this is achieved by ensuring competencies and confidence in skills
● clinical audit.

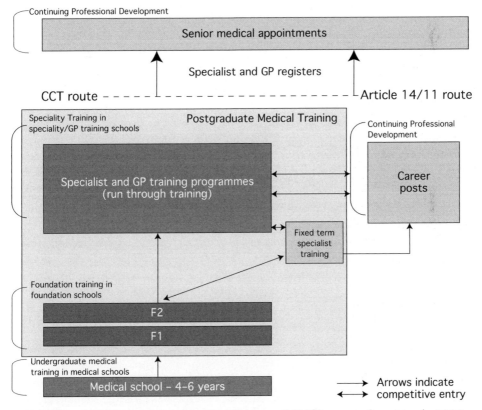

FIGURE 8.1 UK Modernising Medical Careers (MMC) career framework, 2006

The MMC guidance has led to trainee-centred learning; therefore you are more in charge of your own career. The advantage of this is that you will know what you are doing each day. To guide you through your training you will have an educational supervisor. It is not intended that the supervisor will tell you what you should be doing, rather be there to help you if you have any concerns and to provide feedback and advice when necessary.

Another advantage of changes in training brought about by the MMC is that you will be able to experience a much wider and particular range of specialties. Specifically, experience in primary care is available much earlier and more readily than ever before. This reflects the large proportion of health service provision occurring within the community. In addition, areas previously neglected, such as academic medicine and research, will become more accessible. However, because the length of training schemes has been shortened you will have less time to make your career choices. Do not worry that you will be left stranded not knowing what you should be doing to get where you want to be. You should also now be encouraged by much better career support throughout your training, as this is an area specifically addressed in the MMC initiative.

WHAT HAS HAPPENED SINCE MMC?

The PMETB states that changes within postgraduate medical education and training have had to occur as a result of changing:[5]
- social demographics (e.g. patient expectations, increasing burden from chronic conditions and multiple comorbidities)
- trainees' needs and expectations (e.g. resulting gender shifts, desire for improved work-life balance)
- political and health services (e.g. introduction of the European Working Time Directive, service needs and targets).

MMC was criticised for making trainees decide what specialty they would like to specialise in too early and being too rigid, making changing specialties difficult. In addition, the 2007 Medical Training Application System (MTAS) was one of a number of implementation fiascos that arose when MMC was made fully operational. Junior doctors were becoming disillusioned that the right people were not getting the right jobs and that many people were not getting jobs at all on the first round of recruitment. This instigated a huge review of postgraduate training structures and application to programmes: the Tooke Report.

THE TOOKE REPORT

Aspiring to Excellence, the final report of the independent inquiry into MMC undertaken by Sir John Tooke, provided recommendations regarding the restructuring and alteration of implementation of postgraduate medical training.[6] Some of the recommendations in the report are UK-wide, others will require responses from each of the four UK countries individually with subsequent partnership. Although it is a long document, it is worth at least skim-reading to familiarise yourself with the content and the areas of training and implementation of training that may be changing over the forthcoming years as well as the reasons underlying these changes.

Amongst many other recommendations the Tooke Report has suggested that:[6]
- medical schools should play a greater role in careers advice
- the employment linkage between Foundation Year 1 and 2 should be broken and Foundation Year 2 should be incorporated into the first year of Core Specialty Training
- ways in which a more flexible approach to the European Working Time Directive could be embraced (*see* Chapter 13)
- overseas students graduating from UK medical schools should be eligible for postgraduate training, as should refugee doctors with the right to remain in the UK
- there should be opportunities for medical management training during postgraduate training.

At the time of print, changes resulting from the Tooke Report have not yet been agreed. They are likely to be extensive; however, due to lessons learnt previously, they are probably also likely to be implemented over a relatively long time-frame. The Department of Health has defined the underlying principles of all changes resulting from the Tooke Report as being:[7]
- focused on quality (e.g. training and career pathways should offer the appropriate depth and breadth of knowledge and experience)
- patient centred (e.g. skills required for listening, understanding and responding to patient needs should be incorporated into education and training programmes)
- clinically driven (e.g. clinicians will be involved in the development and delivery of education and training)
- flexible (e.g. importance is attached to life-long learning)
- valuing people (e.g. education, training and career pathways should be sensitive to trainees' needs)
- promoting life-long learning (e.g. staff need opportunities to continuously update their skills).

MEDICAL EDUCATION ENGLAND

At the time of writing, in response to the Tooke Report, all postgraduate medical education in England may fall under the supervision of the newly formed independent advisory board NHS Medical Education England (NHS:MEE). NHS:MEE, chaired by an independent doctor,[7] will be responsible for co-ordinating reforms of the postgraduate training pathway for doctors.[7] This will include looking at recruitment methods into the Foundation Programme.[7] The underlying principles of the development of NHS:MEE would be to ensure that policy, professional and service perspectives are integrated into the curricula and to safeguard ring-fenced medical education and training budgets.[8] It should also encourage the cohesion of postgraduate deanery activities,[9] including liaison with bodies in devolved countries.[7] Further details regarding NHS:MEE and similar organisations for devolved nations were not available at the time of print.

You are strongly encouraged to read the Department of Health's document, which is referenced heavily in this section: *A High Quality Workforce: NHS next stage review* as this clearly outlines the plans for future reforms and the multiple functions of NHS:MEE.[7]

CURRENT STATUS OF MEDICAL PATHWAYS AND LIKELY AREAS FOR CHANGE

Figure 8.2 demonstrates the postgraduate training pathway as it currently stands and that suggested in the Tooke Report. A tremendous amount of consultation among

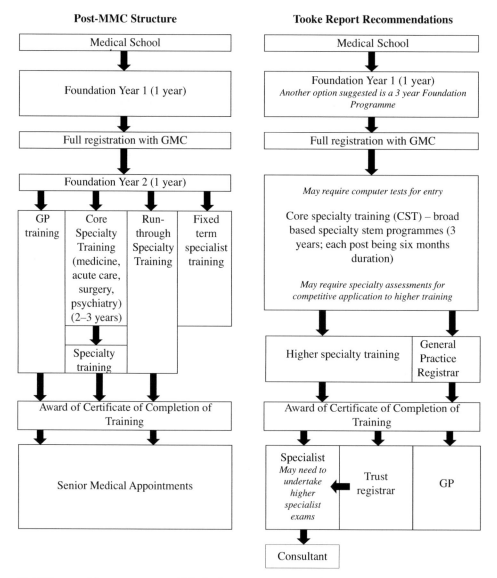

FIGURE 8.2 The current and likely future structure of postgraduate training[5-7]

a plethora of relevant associations, organisations and professional groups has been undertaken before, during and following the Tooke Report. The responses must all be considered, and the solution that best fits all, at the time of print, has not yet been announced. The reforms of the postgraduate training pathways are likely to occur over three years, starting from 2008;[7] only once all this is complete will we know for sure what the pathways will look like.

In addition to altering the pathways for postgraduate training, changes inspired by the Tooke Report will also include the integration of training in leadership, management and teaching for all junior doctors.[7] A clear illustration of the increasing interest in developing clinical managers is shown through the development of BAMMbino, a network of junior doctors who see medical management and leadership as being an intrinsic part of their future career.[10]

You should make sure you keep yourself well up to date with the changes through visiting the MMC website (www.mmc.nhs.uk), royal college websites (*see* Appendix 6), the Foundation Programme website (www.foundationprogramme.nhs. uk) and, when it is launched, the Medical Education England website.

For jobs commencing in 2008 there were both run-through (coupled) and uncoupled specialty posts available. Once trainees have been appointed, and providing they meet all required standards, they will progress to receive their Certificate of Completion of Training (CCT); this is known as 'coupled specialties'. Uncoupled specialties appoint trainees to Core Training, or early years of Specialty Training. These posts do not guarantee progression to CCT as trainees are required to competitively reapply to higher years of Specialty Training. If the postgraduate training pathways are altered as per Tooke's recommendation, the uncoupled template may be implemented more broadly, as all trainees will undertake Core Specialty Training before entering the specialty stream of their choice at Higher Specialist Training level. However, there is some reluctance to adopt this template in a blanket fashion across all specialties.[11] Coupled and uncoupled specialties, as they were for the 2008 recruitment round, are demonstrated in Table 8.1.

TABLE 8.1 Coupled and uncoupled specialties, correct for recruitment for August 2008

Coupled	Uncoupled
Paediatrics	Core medical training
General practice	Acute care common stem
Radiology	Core surgical training
Pathology	Core psychiatric training
Obstetrics and gynaecology	Anaesthetics
Public health	
Neurosurgery	
Ophthalmology	

Specific and/or procedural changes following implementation of the recommendations of the Tooke Report are also likely to include:[6,9]

- limited ability to move between programmes during the Core Specialty Training (CST)
- CST is likely to have a small number of stems (e.g. medical specialties, surgical specialties, community specialties and/or GP, diagnostic specialties and acute common stem)[12]
- a short period of time in general practice will be incorporated in the majority of CST rotations
- staff grade level is retained and allows doctors to undertake career posts below CCT level if they cannot or do not want to progress to Higher Specialty Training
- general practice training will increase from three years' to five years' duration
- academic clinical fellowships (*see* Chapter 16) are likely to slot in at the Higher Specialist Training level.

At the time of writing, an issue that remains unclear is exactly how the academic clinical training fits in with the new model of postgraduate training. It is most likely to coincide with the Higher Specialty Training phase, but this is yet to be announced.

REFERENCES

1 Modernising Medical Careers. *Rough Guide: Foundation years*, 2005. Available at: www. foundationprogramme.nhs.uk/pages/foundation-doctors/key-documents#rough-guide-to-the-foundation-programme (accessed 8 February 2009).

2 MacDonald R. Modernising Medical Careers. *StudentBMJ*. 2003; **11**: 372–3.

3 Department of Health. *Modernising Medical Careers: the next steps*. London: Department of Health; 2004.

4 Department of Health. *New training programme heralds in a new era in UK medicine*. London: Department of Health; 2005. Available at www.dh.gov.uk/en/Publicationsandstatistics/Press releases/DH_4107657 (accessed 8 February 2009).

5 Postgraduate Medical Education and Training Board. PMETB Briefing 002. *Educating Tomorrow's Doctors: challenges for the future*. London: Postgraduate Medical Education and Training Board; 2008. Available at: www.pmetb.org.uk (accessed 13 January 2009).

6 Tooke J. *Aspiring to Excellence: findings and final recommendations of the independent inquiry into modernising medical careers*. London: MMC Inquiry; 2008. Available at: www.mmcinquiry.org. uk/Final_8_Jan_08_MMC_all.pdf (accessed 13 January 2009).

7 Department of Health. *A High Quality Workforce: NHS next stage review*. London: Department of Health; 2008.

8 Newshound. *BMJ Careers*. 2008; **337**: 2.

9 Department of Health. *The Secretary of State for Health's Response to Aspiring to Excellence: final report of the independent inquiry into modernising medical careers*. London: Department of Health; 2008.

10 www.bamm.co.uk/Services/Support_&_Development/BAMMbino_2007072440/

11 Secretary of State for Health. *The Government Response to the Health Select Committee Report 'Modernising Medical Careers'*. Norwich: The Stationery Office; 2008.

12 Delamothe T. Tooke's take on what went wrong with MMC. *BMJ Careers*. 2008: **20**–1.

FURTHER READING

Conference of Postgraduate Medical Deans of the United Kingdom. Available at: www.copmed.org.uk (accessed 13 January 2009). This includes, among other things, links to many career-related and institution websites.

9

The Foundation Programme

The Foundation Programme was launched in full for doctors starting work in August 2005. It is designed to bridge the gap between undergraduate and specialist medical training.[1] This chapter will explain what the Foundation Programme is, how it is delivered, what the expectations of Foundation doctors are and how you will be assessed.

WHAT IS THE FOUNDATION PROGRAMME?[1,2]

In 1953, following the Goodenough Report,[1] the PRHO year (the first year as a doctor following graduation from medical school) was introduced as part of medical training to enable application of knowledge and a widening of the new doctor's experience. This was expected to occur with the support of guidance and supervision. In 1975, the PRHO year was criticised by the Merrison Report,[1] which found that it had inadequate organisation, definition of aims and understanding of the proper interaction of the service and education. These issues remained a problem until recently. Part of the reason for this was that the PRHO year had changed very little since its introduction nearly half a century earlier. Therefore the Foundation Programme was designed to address these issues and was launched, in full, for all new doctors who started work in August 2005. To ensure that the Foundation Programme met adequate standards of training the curriculum was agreed with the GMC and the PMETB.

By placing the onus of completion of objectives on you, the trainee, rather than the trainer, the Foundation Programme has made the first year post-graduation. Competency is established in a structured way through the use of standardised assessments and structured supervision. This type of trainee-led programme equips you with the skills necessary to manage your professional development in the future.

Currently Foundation Year 1 (F1) and Foundation Year 2 (F2) make up the current two-year Foundation Programme, which all UK medical graduates are required to undertake before progressing to specialty or GP training. The Foundation Programme usually consists of six, four-month attachments.

However, it may be delivered in six-month blocks. Usually the F1 year will consist of at least three months of medicine and three months of surgical experience. Obviously the delivery of the Foundation Programme may change as a result of the Tooke Report; however, the duration of posts and requirement to have experience of particular specialties are likely to remain the same.

You will also have protected 'bleep-free' time for planned learning. F2 is equivalent to the first year of the old-style senior house officer (SHO) post, in which you can build upon the skills and knowledge you acquired in F1. As with the pre-Foundation training, you will receive provisional registration from the GMC upon graduation and you will qualify for full GMC registration after successful completion of the F1 year. Although true at the time of printing, this may change in favour of an outcome-based programme for which successful completion would be required before full registration may take place. If this were to go ahead, provisional registration would occur at the same time, but full registration may occur anywhere between graduation and completion of Foundation training. The current situation is that all medical graduates are required to complete the Foundation Programme in order to work as doctors in the UK.

So, what are the general expectations of you during your Foundation Programme? Although it is a bridge to your future, the following are expected. You should be:
- able to put your knowledge, skills and attitudes, learnt at medical school, into practice
- gaining new knowledge and skills; a particular focus of the Foundation Programme is acquisition of the skills required to recognise and manage acutely ill patients
- fine-tuning your professional attitudes.

Completion of the Foundation Programme requires you to demonstrate progress in the standards set out by the GMC in a document called *The New Doctor* (*see* Chapter 11). Assessments used are described in full at www.foundationprogramme. nhs.uk; however, they include the following.
- Multi-source feedback (there are two tools in use, dependent on the deanery at which you are training):
  - mini-peer assessment tool (mini-PAT) – you will have to nominate eight assessors from your team, nursing staff or allied health professional colleagues to fill out a questionnaire that is returned anonymously; you will also have to complete a self-assessment using the same questionnaire
  - team assessment of behaviour (TAB) – you will have to select 10 co-workers to assess you using 360° TAB forms with envelopes addressed to the Foundation Training Programme Director (FTPD) to enable anonymous return of the form.
- Direct observation of doctor–patient interaction:
  - mini-clinical evaluation exercise (mini-CEX) – a 15-minute observed encounter with a patient in order to assess your clinical skills, attitudes, behaviours and ability to provide good patient care
  - direct observation of procedural skills (DOPS) – a structured checklist to assess your practical skills.
- Case-based discussion (CBD) – a structured discussion with your supervisor about a clinical case you are involved in to establish your clinical reasoning and judgement skills.

So what can you expect to be doing during your Foundation training? The British Medical Association 2006 cohort study revealed the common tasks of F1 doctors as including: prescribing, ordering and checking investigations, routine filing and paperwork, inserting intravenous cannula, taking bloods, clerking cases, and diagnosing conditions. Less common, but still regular, jobs included participating in elective surgery (when in an appropriate post), administration of intravenous drugs and recording ECGs. Apart from some activities (e.g. participating in elective surgery), the regularity with which F1 doctors undertake the above activities followed the same trend across medicine, surgical and 'other' placements.[1] Therefore, do not be too concerned if your Foundation placements are not exactly the ones you would like as you will probably all be learning the same skills. If you do want to have experience of a particular specialty you can try to arrange a taster experience (*see* Chapter 10) or undertaking audits in your desired specialty.

All Foundation trainees are expected to undertake appraisals at the beginning and end of every post. A mid-post appraisal is also recommended, but is not compulsory. It is a useful experience so you are strongly recommended to undertake your mid-post appraisal if possible. It is crucial that you utilise this time to maximum effect as your appraisals are the key to your training within that post. The Foundation Programme portfolio available from the Foundation Programme website (www. foundationprogramme.nhs.uk) contains templates for appraisal topics to be addressed as part of your appraisal; in addition your e-portfolio will contain relevant material. However, some deaneries provide their trainees with their own appraisal booklets also. The cornerstone of your appraisal and learning is the personal development plan (PDP), in to which you, along with your educational supervisor, should work out your weak areas (your 'learning needs') and how you will tackle these throughout the post. Try to enter realistic needs as well as achievable and measurable ways of meeting them. For example, if your learning need is breaking bad news, you can tackle this through observation of colleagues doing this, reading up on the theory of how this is best done then doing it yourself, initially under observation of seniors. A measurable way of knowing if you have achieved this is through successful completion of a mini-CEX.

Trainees are required to complete a reflective diary. This ensures that you learn from both bad and good experiences, no matter how big or small they are. There are example reflection sheets in Appendices 4 and 5; you may also have templates within an e-portfolio/portfolio. Although many people struggle with this and/or feel it is a waste of time, you can use your reflective practice to direct your learning, instigate discussion with colleagues and to help you to update/develop your PDP. On a more superficial basis, if you regularly undertake reflection and maintain a reflective diary you will find job applications much easier in the future as many of the white box questions on job application forms can be answered directly from cases you will reflect upon.

Following successful completion of the Foundation Programme, you will receive a Foundation Achievement of Competency Document (FACD), which you require in order to enter Specialty Training positions.

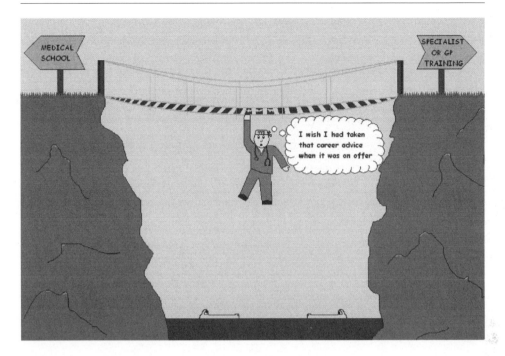

POSTGRADUATE DEANERIES AND FOUNDATION SCHOOLS

The UK has been divided up geographically into 'deaneries'. A postgraduate dean heads each deanery and each deanery has responsibility for the delivery of the Foundation Programme training in its area, through Foundation schools. A Foundation school is not the same as a postgraduate medical school. It does not represent a building but a number of institutions grouped together to offer the required variety of placements to ensure complete and wide education and training. Within a Foundation school there will be acute and mental health trusts, general practices, universities and other relevant institutions, such as hospices and public health departments (*see* Figure 9.1).

Specifically, each deanery must ensure that the standards set by the GMC and the PMETB are being met. The deaneries in the UK are:

- East Midlands Healthcare Workforce
- East of England
- Kent, Sussex and Surrey
- London
- Mersey
- Northern
- Northern Ireland
- North Western
- Oxford
- Scotland (divided into East, West, North and South-East regions)
- Severn Institute
- South West Peninsula

- South Yorkshire and South Humber
- Wales
- Wessex
- West Midlands Workforce
- Yorkshire and the Humber Postgraduate.

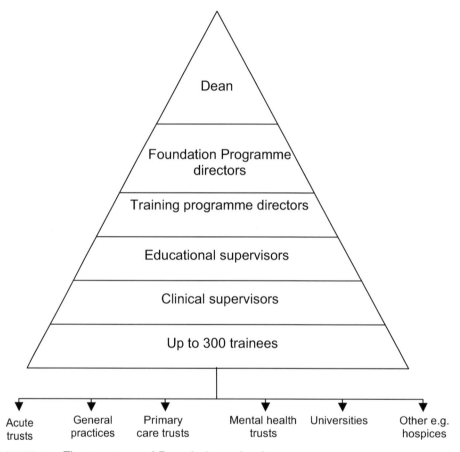

FIGURE 9.1 The structure of Foundation schools

You should obtain up-to-date information from the COPMED website (www. copmed.org.uk/contacts/).

It is important that you familiarise yourself with the roles of a postgraduate deanery, which include:

- provision of information about and recruitment to the Foundation Programme
- arranging shadowing and/or induction periods prior to starting F1 (*see* Chapter 10 for more information on shadowing periods)
- establishing that local assessment procedures are in accordance with national procedures
- ensuring that regular and appropriate appraisals occur

- ensuring that those undertaking assessments receive adequate training
- provision of appropriate career management and development opportunities and advice to enable a smooth progression of trainees from F1 to F2 including assistance in gaining taster experiences.

Occasionally Foundation trainees need to change deaneries once they have begun their training. There are very specific eligibility criteria for doing this, which include significant family responsibilities, chronic illness or disability requiring local follow-up or terminally ill first-degree relative. For full information on the eligibility criteria and the processes of inter-deanery transfer see the *Foundation School Transfers Guidance Notes and Process* section on the Foundation Programme website (www. foundationprogramme.nhs.uk).

REFERENCES

1 British Medical Association. *The Cohort Study of 2006 Medical Graduates*. 2nd report. London: British Medical Association; 2008.
2 General Medical Council. *The New Doctor: recommendations on general clinical training*. 2005. Available at: www.gmc-uk.org/education/postgraduate/new_doctor.asp (accessed 8 February 2009).
3 Modernising Medical Careers. *Frequently Asked Questions*. Available at: www.foundation programme.nhs.uk/pages/home/faqs (accessed 13 January 2009).

FURTHER READING

British Medical Association. *Guidance on Applying for Foundation Programmes*. London: British Medical Association; 2005.
British Medical Association Medical Education Sub-committee of the Board of Science. *Medical Specialties: the way forward*. London: British Medical Association; 2007.
Shahin YA. Have you filled in the assessment forms? *BMJ Careers*. 2007; **334**: 65–6.
www.foundationprogramme.nhs.uk

10

Broadening your clinical experience

The medical school curriculum is designed so that you can choose what you want to study at certain times. This chapter highlights the parts of your course that give you the freedom to decide what you want to study and how you can make best use of these times.

Broadening your clinical experience with focused placements has the potential to support you in making informed and appropriate decisions about your career development early on in your training.[1] The best way to decide whether or not you enjoy a particular aspect of medicine is to experience it first-hand. There are many opportunities to sample various aspects of medicine within your course, including student-selected components, your elective and intercalated degrees (where available and should you choose to do one). Other opportunities also exist outside your course, such as part-time jobs, summer jobs, work experience and specialty courses. During your Foundation years some deaneries also allow you to sample additional career alternatives ('tasters') in other areas of medicine for a few days at a time. However, you may have to use your study leave entitlement to do this. You will have to write a report on your time in that specialty, which includes the skills that would be required, in addition to the ones you possess, to succeed in that specialty.

You may want to use these optional components of your curriculum to do the following.

- Fill in the deficiencies in your course as well as learning about the subjects inadequately covered to address your learning needs. For example, many medical courses do not allow time for specialist areas such as ear, nose and throat (ENT), ophthalmology, dermatology or A&E, and you may wish to use your time to sample them.
- Broaden areas of interest that can apply to any career, such as academic placements and other areas you may wish to know more about.
- Follow any particular interests (but try to remain open-minded).

STUDENT-SELECTED COMPONENTS

Student-selected components (SSCs), or student-selected modules (SSMs) as they are known in some universities, were created in 1993 following the GMC publication *Tomorrow's Doctors*,[2] which recommended that students should be allowed to follow their own interests beyond the curriculum. SSCs were designed to allow students to study a particular area of interest in more depth. Some medical schools allow you to take one or more SSCs abroad as well as your elective. You could pursue new interests, develop existing ones or provide experience that is relevant to the preceding, or a future, main module:

> 'I chose an SSC module in A&E at the Royal Shrewsbury Hospital. It was a great chance to develop my basic skills, gain confidence in speaking and eliciting histories, as well as developing an understanding of symptom differentials. This attachment also allowed me to become independent in my thinking with respect to investigations and management of patients. I saw a variety of medicine and was able to develop and further my knowledge.' (Janaki Gnananandha, third-year medical student, Keele University.)

Medical schools deliver SSCs in different ways. SSCs may encompass between two and five weeks at different points throughout your medical studies from Year 1 onwards. SSCs in the clinical years usually become more clinically oriented and self-directed.[3]

SSCs can be medical, clinical, managerial, a project or research-based. They can also be non-medical but remain medically related. These include the history of medicine, medicine art, modern languages, music or sign language, complementary and alternative medicine, sports medicine, radiology, journalism, arts, humanities and even medical career support. You could also choose to work with the police, take part in scientific and community projects (Manchester), become involved in medical publishing (Oxford) or study shiatsu and yoga (Peninsula). The possibilities are endless. Although a list of options and placements is often held by the university, now that you have read about the many different types of SSC on offer, how about proposing your own?

Students are usually allocated places on a one-to-one or a two-to-one basis to a consultant supervisor. How the student spends that time is entirely for negotiation between student and supervisor. It is worth noting that, apart from your own personal aims and learning objectives for the SSC, your university may have others in mind for each of these aspects of your course. For example, at East Anglia the aims of SSCs fall into two parts:[3]

- to assess a student's ability to gather, appraise and present information within a set list of domains
- to learn how to review and appraise research papers, assessed through a formal written appraisal for every unit.

Thus, SSCs may test a student's ability to:[4]

- gather data by questionnaire and/or oral interview
- use library and information services to perform literature searches
- gather data from the literature and critically evaluate it as well as ranking the range and level of authority of different forms of scientific literature
- compile information into a written report that addresses the topic to be investigated
- use computer technology to compile and submit a written report and be able to deliver an oral presentation.

Other learning objectives may include how you demonstrate:[4]
- achievement of the specific objectives originally set
- appreciation of the legal and personal needs to respect confidentiality and/or sensitive issues relating to human subjects
- reflection of how you have worked with other healthcare professionals
- in-depth knowledge of one particular subject including, if appropriate, public health aspects, prevention, epidemiology, treatment options and future development in relation to one or more patients.

The best thing you can do at the start of your SSC is to determine what objectives you and your university are setting so that you know how to meet them.

Your assessment may include your written report of the case, the oral presentation, workbook, poster presentation or written examination. Your attendance is also taken into account as well as your performance against the learning objectives agreed between yourself and your supervisor.

In the article *Getting the most out of your SSMs*,[5] students were asked about their opinions and experiences of SSCs. Some sensible top tips were:
- start early
- read information carefully and e-mail tutors to clarify details
- think about how much time you want to, or can, give a placement
- only request choices you want – you cannot guarantee you will get your first choice
- do not be put off by people attempting to stop you doing what you want
- do something you will enjoy and that will also further your medical education
- find a tutor who shares your special interest – the more interested your tutor is and the more interested you are the more you will gain from completing the SSC
- do something original
- go into your SSC with an open mind
- do not be disheartened; your fifth choice could be just as rewarding – you will often find, even if you have not been given your first-choice SSC, that so long as you 'get into' your project you will probably end up enjoying it
- do not waste it.

ELECTIVE

The elective is an integral part of the medical course and is usually a period of between 8 and 12 weeks taken as a continuous block of study. It is often seen as a major highlight of the time spent at medical school.

The timing of the elective depends on the university, but it is usually scheduled during clinical studies so that you already have a good broad base in order to maximise your learning. It is an invaluable learning resource and not a holiday, though a holiday can be, and often is, added on.

Think what you want to achieve

> 'I did my elective at St John's Medical College Hospital in Bangalore, India. I chose this as it is a charity and privately run hospital in a large city in India, and I saw the elective as an opportunity to throw myself into a completely different culture in a country I knew very little about yet which is rich in diversity in terms of places to visit and the people that live there. From my experience, I learnt that very different factors influence healthcare in India compared to the UK, largely religion and costs! I also had the opportunity to explore cities, mountains, national parks and beaches – experiencing the Hindi culture and Indian way of life at first hand. All in all, an amazing eight weeks.' (Gemma Cooper-Hobson, final-year medical student at Manchester University [Keele cohort])

As it is a period of self-directed learning, many students choose to go overseas, taking the chance to see non-NHS medicine and to experience the practice of medicine in an unfamiliar setting where the scientific, social, economic or cultural standards are different. There are very diverse healthcare systems across the globe, from the underdeveloped third-world hospitals where you may get a lot of 'hands on' experience, to the ultra modern and high-tech institutes where you may see ground-breaking procedures. Or, instead of practising your clinical skills, how about electing to teach in Tanzania, like four medical students from University College London did?[6] The opportunities are endless; depending on your learning needs, interests and what you want to achieve. It is what you make of it.

Research, research, research

You have to organise your elective yourself, which means you can apply wherever you wish. Unfortunately, there are scams out there so be careful if money is being asked for in advance. Make sure your supervisor is medically qualified and that you are not putting yourself at undue risk. Also make sure you start planning your elective early. The most popular electives are often taken up years in advance and the application procedure for some can be extremely complex and time consuming. In view of political instability in some areas, you should be aware of the safety issues and check about countries you intend to visit on the Foreign & Commonwealth Office website (www.fco.gov.uk). You should recheck this advice just before leaving for your elective as political situations can change rapidly. The elective co-ordinators at your medical school may help if you have to change your plans suddenly because of such an event.

There are a lot of resources that provide information on electives to help with your choices. *The Medic's Guide to Work and Electives Around the World*[7] is a very user-friendly and informative manual. (If you prefer web-based information visit www.medicstravel.co.uk) This is a phenomenal resource that includes a plethora of information on hospitals across the globe. It has useful travel tips for those of you planning to work or take an elective abroad. In addition, for an administrative fee, *Medics Travel* provides a service to help you plan your elective. UK and Irish medical students who are members of the Medical Defence Union (MDU) also have access to the *Electives Network*.[8] This resource was designed to provide elective planning information and thus contains information on what you need to consider when planning your elective as well details of over 100 popular elective destinations and over 5000 hospitals and medical schools. The site also provides feedback and articles about the experiences of medical students who have already taken their elective.

Speak to others

Some universities may provide a copy of addresses used by students in previous years, may have existing arrangements with international institutions, or may have student-led exchange programmes. Speak to previous elective students, doctors and consultants on the wards, and find out what they did and what they would not do now. Some universities also keep elective reports.

Be prepared

Make sure when choosing a place, that you research the health and working conditions there.

The National Travel Health Network and Centre website (www.nathnac.org/travel/index.htm) provides advice on aspects of travel health from insect bite avoidance through to travellers' diarrhoea. There are multiple information sheets that can be downloaded from the website providing information on non-infectious and infectious health risks. Visit the Country Information pages to get advice on the health information you require and details of some of the relevant health risks for the country(ies) you will be visiting. Useful information regarding accessing healthcare when you are abroad can be obtained at www.nhs.uk/Healthcareabroad/Pages/Healthcareabroad.aspx

Sort out your vaccinations and HIV prophylaxis well in advance; there should be contacts at your medical school who can advise you on these. You should also make sure that your travel insurance covers you. There are some travel insurance policies specifically for medical students on their elective. It is worth researching these. Accommodation may be arranged for you, but you must check this is the case. Extra bursaries are available to help with this (*see* 'Money matters' below).

Important information about travel arrangements

Some students have found themselves in trouble on their elective. If you are going abroad check the expiry date on your passport, as some countries require you to have at least six months left at the date of your return.

Check whether you need a visa and if you do, ensure it is the correct one. Allow plenty of time for this to be processed. The Foreign & Commonwealth Office website travel advice section provides useful advice on visas and other requirements.

You will not usually require a work permit visa as you are not being paid and you do not usually require a student study visa, hence, you should apply for a normal visitor's visa unless your host university or hospital instructs you otherwise. Always check this out before setting off on your travels.

Insurance and malpractice cover

Universities usually do *not* insure you against malpractice and for health cover whilst you are on your elective. Contact the MDU, Medical and Dental Defence Union of Scotland (MDDUS), Medical Protection Society (MPS) or any other medical defence organisation, to arrange insurance cover when travelling abroad on your elective.

If you are applying to North America, Canada or Israel you must enquire about malpractice cover. The MPS, MDU and MDDUS (free abroad) will help in the USA. The host university may make arrangements for you or the host university may direct you as to how you can obtain it. You will almost certainly have to pay for insurance cover in North America and the amounts vary. In Canada and Israel, insurance is usually arranged for you, but again you will often have to pay.

The MDU has produced a useful guide on your elective placement, including malpractice cover. There is more information about medical defence organisations in the section on the roles of important organisations and societies.

Letters of recommendation

Letters of recommendation are not routinely provided for applicants for electives. However, if a letter of recommendation, or a letter to confirm your status as a student, is required in your individual case, your medical school should provide one. Contact your medical school in good time to allow for administration.

Money matters

Unfortunately, you will have to pay for your elective. Electives can be expensive, though it really does depend on what you want to do. There are numerous grants, awards, research awards, sponsorships, bursaries and prizes available. If you are well-organised you can get a considerable amount of support, although it is easier if you are incorporating some research into your elective, as most awards and grants are awarded in exchange for some sort of project report or research work. Grants and awards are sometimes offered as part of a competition, particularly if the elective is related to the professional body or organisation offering the money. Previously, awards and prizes have been on offer from the Wellcome Trust, MDDUS, and MDU. The BMA holds a list of organisations to which you can apply for funding. Information on research and development funding can also be found at www.rdinfo. org.uk. Currently, the database holds information from more than 1300 funding bodies, offering over 5000 different awards.

And now for something different

If you decide to stay in the same country as your medical school, do something useful or different with your time. How about getting involved in medical politics, a project at an academic or a pharmaceutical research centre or even working with the team doctor at a football club? Remember some of your peers, with whom you will be competing for Foundation places in the near future, will be off working with Tibetan monks in Lhasa's community hospital[9] or in the Gambia assisting a voluntary service overseas' paediatrician.[10] So try to be original and find something interesting and stimulating to do in your home country.

INTERCALATED DEGREES

Intercalated degrees[3] are usually one-year degree courses that can be undertaken during a year away from your medical degree in a variety of subjects related to medicine, and they provide an opportunity to pursue further study in an area of interest. In some universities students are allowed to study for the extra degree within other faculties of the university or at other institutes or universities. Consider doing this if you have a particular interest that cannot be fulfilled at your medical school, if your interest is in a very popular and oversubscribed subject or if a particular university is renowned for a research interest that appeals to you.[11]

Interest in intercalated degrees has grown over the years as they allow you to study a particular area of interest in greater depth. They enable you to gain valuable skills in either clinical, laboratory or epidemiological research.[11]

You can obtain a Bachelor of Science (BSc), Bachelor of Medical Science (BMedSci), Bachelor of Arts (BA) or you can do a Masters in Medical Science (MMedSc) for an additional year of study. Such degrees are commonly undertaken once you have completed at least two years of study as a medical student, hence, after Year 2 or Year 3, though entry policies differ at different universities.

Traditionally, in some institutions, intercalated degrees were only open to high flyers. You would have had to have passed all your exams and not repeated a year, to be considered. In some medical schools allocation is by invitation only, but this is slowly changing. Allocation, however, may still be on a competitive basis. In other universities, intercalated degrees are not only open to any student, but actively encouraged. Figures show that between 20% and 40% of medical students intercalate.[11] In medical schools where intercalated degrees are voluntary, as many as 50% of each year group intercalate at some point in their studies.[3] At some universities intercalating degrees are compulsory.

Degrees may be awarded in research- or library-based projects. They can be medical as well as social science degrees. Biological sciences subjects you may be able to study include:

- anthropology
- psychology
- anatomy
- biochemistry
- cell biology
- physiology
- microbiology
- pharmacology
- medical or molecular genetics
- neuroscience
- pathology
- laboratory-based research project

- sports medicine
- forensic archaeology
- space physiology.

Degrees in integrated health science subjects are fewer in number and include:
- public health
- ethics and law
- behavioural science
- history of medicine
- management.

The main consideration in extending the already lengthy medical course is that you will need to finance 12 additional months. Fees may be payable for the year, but in some institutes separate funding may be available. At some universities tuition fees for this year are paid, but you need to pay living costs. Find out about this before embarking on such a degree.

Intercalated degrees are thought to result in better study habits with higher 'deep' and 'strategic' learning scores.[12] They are also thought to be particularly useful if you are considering a career in research or academic medicine or teaching as a career. It is an opportunity to derive potentially publishable original research project material and have chance to publish papers, which adds weight to your CV.[13]

To gain maximum benefit from your intercalated degree you should aim to pass it with as high a grade as possible. In certain scoring systems for job applications only degrees awarded with higher classes will be taken into consideration; this is especially true if you have undertaken a compulsory intercalated degree.

Intercalated Degree Student Profile

Name: Sam Creavin

Year of intercalation: Between Year 4 and 5

Intercalated degree: MPhil in Epidemiology

Medical School: Keele University School of Medicine, Manchester Curriculum

Institution at which intercalated degree undertaken: Keele University

Why do an intercalated degree: I thought intercalating would aid my personal development and be a bit different from the standard undergraduate course.

How did you choose your intercalated degree: I wanted to learn about research and methodology in general rather than about one thing (such as anatomy) in more depth. The MPhil met these objectives.

Benefits: I've spent most of the year conducting my own original research as well as attending masters level modules in research methods, epidemiology and statistics. I believe I find, read and understand research papers much faster and that I'm now more able to conduct future research or audits. These skills will help me to practise evidence-based medicine, which will, in turn, improve the care I give to patients. The increased flexibility in my time has allowed me to take on more extra-curricular activities.

Downsides: The extra year is expensive. As well as the cost of the year you're ultimately losing one year of your final salary. It's hard to see your peers in your old year go on and graduate.

Advice to a student considering intercalating: Like anything, there's no point in doing it just for your CV; you should have a real interest in your chosen topic. Think about what you want to do, and consider looking at other medical schools if there isn't something offered by your own. Plan ahead as application for funding is competitive and the deadlines are easy to miss. Set your learning objectives for the year at the start and regularly assess your progress. Try to use the increased flexibility in your time to develop other interests. I've also had ad hoc days in the hospital to maintain my clinical competence, and I'd recommend that.

EUROPEAN EXCHANGE PROGRAMMES

The International Federation of Medical Students' Association (IFMSA) is an international exchange scheme that allows medical students from across the world to literally swap places for a few weeks. This allows them to complete a clinical attachment in a range of over 70 countries; the exchange scheme is huge. In Europe, the scheme involves Malta, Italy, Estonia and Germany. For terms and conditions and frequently asked questions visit the website (www.ifmsa.org).[5]

The European Community Action Scheme for the Mobility of University Students (ERASMUS) was set up in 1987. It provides organisation and funding to enable university students of any discipline to take part in an exchange with another European country during part of their course.[14] In the minority of medical schools, these schemes allow you to study a foreign language and complete a period of study abroad. You usually spend up to three months (although it could be up to a year depending on the university) at various places in Europe, including France, Germany and Scandinavia. The exact amount of time, year of placement and location depend on your university and the links that it has in place; practices vary considerably between universities. There is also less emphasis on practising clinical medicine than there is with the elective. Contact your ERASMUS head at your university for details on availability of and information about your local ERASMUS schemes.

SUMMER JOBS AND PART-TIME WORK

Although part-time work during term time is often discouraged by medical schools due to the challenging and demanding nature of the course and the amount of study needed, it is often a necessity and many students have managed to get through the course with a part-time job. Try to find something that has potential to be flexible (e.g. around examination time) and that only requires you to work in the evenings or at weekends. If you are already working, re-evaluate your situation when you think your job may start affecting your university work and not when it actually does.

So what can you do? Well, anything really. As well as casual work in bars and restaurants carried out by students of other subjects, many medical students choose to work as healthcare assistants, medical secretaries in hospitals or note summarisers in general practices. These medical-related jobs can usually be arranged through your teaching hospital, other local hospitals or via GPs that take medical students on attachments, all of which would be on file at your medical school. There are also nursing agencies or nurse banks that you can sign up to directly. Although working for a nurse bank or agency has the drawback that work is not guaranteed, it has the huge benefit that to some extent you can choose when and where you want to work as you can decline shifts that are not convenient to you.

Try to find a job that will not only earn you extra money, but also can be used in future job applications as evidence that you have spent time preparing yourself for becoming a doctor. The benefit of you undertaking a part-time job in a role such as a healthcare assistant can be mutually beneficial to both your learning and your employer also as not many healthcare assistants have the knowledge of a fourth-year medical student. A few examples of how part-time jobs can provide experience of skills required of a good doctor can be found in Table 10.1.

WORK EXPERIENCE

Work experience is not just the period of time you spend in a clinical environment before entering medical school, it can be useful throughout medical school and your Foundation training. You need to make some big decisions about which specialty you want to spend the rest of your life in. Without really understanding and experiencing what the work in that specialty involves, you will not be able to make an informed decision.

As a medical student it is easy to end up shadowing the Foundation doctors who are undertaking lots of generic administrative jobs, which are no different from specialty to specialty. It is important to gain information on what you should be doing at their stage; however it does not really help to inform you about your long-term career intentions. Shadowing consultants often occurs in ward rounds where time may be limited and patient contact brief, or in clinics, where you only see a certain proportion of the patient population. Therefore, shadowing the senior Specialty Trainees (ST3s or above) whilst on different rotations or GPs on their out-of-hours shifts is of great benefit as it gives you a deeper understanding of the type of work undertaken in that specialty. It is well worth trying to spend a good period of time over different days with the same registrar to get experience of a good mix of both ward, theatre and clinic work (as applicable).

Foundation doctors have a formal structure for 'work experience' as you are offered the opportunity to undertake taster sessions. All foundation trainees are entitled to use up to two weeks of their study leave for taster sessions over the two years providing cover for your clinical duties can be met. This time should be used to undertake a period of experience in a specialty in which you currently have limited experience and want to see if this is a specialty you would like to consider applying to for Specialty Training. A full timetable that ensures you have full involvement with the clinical team should be developed.[15] This opportunity is invaluable if you have not yet had the chance to work in the specialty you are most interested in. Speak with your Foundation Programme Director and/or Educational Supervisor for more information about arranging a taster session. Try to arrange the experience as early as possible in a placement to enable it to occur at the most optimum time for all concerned.

TABLE 10.1 How part-time jobs can provide experience of skills required of a good doctor

Job(s)	Skills learnt in the job associated with being a good doctor
Bar, shop and restaurant work	Communicating with the general public – sometimes in difficult or fraught circumstances
	Responsibility and probity – often you are in charge looking after of money, stock or premises
	Teamwork – especially when at busy times
Babysitting	Communication with young children
	Responsibility – it is a good sign of responsibility if parents feel you are responsible to look after their children
Healthcare assistant	Understanding how the NHS operates – including the constraints and difficulties of this
	Teamwork – multidisciplinary teams
	Building basic medical knowledge
	Learning how to communicate with patients of different ages and with different problems
	Nature and importance of confidentiality and consent
Medical secretaries	Understanding how the NHS operates – including the constraints and difficulties of this
	Building basic medical knowledge
	Learning to communicate with healthcare professionals and the general public
	Nature and importance of confidentiality
GP notes summariser	Exposure to medical problems and how they are managed
	Understanding of how healthcare is provided in primary care
	Understanding of medical coding systems
	Nature and importance of confidentiality
Haematology or pathology laboratory technician	Understand the processes involved in obtaining clinical tests
Phlebotomy	Practising the very useful skill of taking blood
	Communication with patients including obtaining consent for a procedure

VOLUNTEERING

Not everybody is aware of the possibility of volunteering and the infinite number of areas in which you can be a volunteer. Medical students and trainee doctors can be great volunteers due to the vast range of skills they have. However, you must only become a volunteer if you can spare the time and you are truly committed. Do not join a scheme with the sole intention of boosting your CV as this is not fair on the other people involved. Whatever your interest and/or time available there will be a call for volunteers. Here are some examples of local volunteer work you could undertake.

- Help out on a research project – this can benefit you most if you volunteer for a research project that covers an area of interest to you.
- Join your local Red Cross or St John's Ambulance brigade – often this involves once weekly meetings and you can help provide first aid cover at various events, which can range from local plays right through to professional football matches.
- Nursing homes, rest homes or hospitals – volunteers at nursing homes, rest homes and hospitals are sometimes requested to just speak with patients to provide company, run shops or serve teas. This can be a good way of learning to speak with, often elderly, patients as well as benefiting them greatly.
- University work – universities are often looking for students to volunteer to support the running of various events. This can be a good way to meet fellow students and find out more about your university.
- Medical student led charities (e.g. the charity MARROW, part of the Antony Nolan Bone Marrow Trust [www.anthonynolan.org.uk/about/howtogetinvolved/marrow.htm])

You can undertake volunteer work further afield as well. You may wish to organise this yourself by approaching organisations and charities. However, if you want some help, you can approach organisations such as:

- Concordia (www.concordia-iye.org.uk/)
- Community Service Volunteers (www.csv.org.uk)
- MedSin (www.medsin.org)
- Voluntary Services Overseas (www.vso.org.uk)

SPECIALTY COURSES

There are a number of specialty courses, which you may have the opportunity to attend, that allow you to further your knowledge about specific aspects of medicine, for example, for students interested in trauma medicine the Trauma Conference, run by Bart's and the London Queen Mary's School of Medicine, provided lectures covering the airway, breathing, circulation (ABC) principles, head injuries, paediatric emergency medicine and conflict medicine. In addition, there were also extrication demonstrations and practical sessions.[16] At the time of print the London Trauma Conference was available for both medical students and doctors consists of a three-day programme of seminars, master classes, debates and breakaway sessions.[17]

The Royal Society of Medicine also runs over 400 academic meetings, lectures and workshops every year, many of which are free to medical students. There are ample opportunities to further your knowledge in all specialties of medicine as well as if you have a specific field of interest.[18]

PasTest runs a variety courses for medical students, as well as doctors, at various levels in their careers. The company provides over 90 best-selling titles covering all areas of medical revision.[19]

Many short courses are run by medical schools and royal colleges, covering a wide variety of subject matter in various specialties throughout the year. For instance, the Royal College of General Practitioners has a series of courses held across the UK on many educational subjects (e.g. skin problems, drug and substance misuse and mental health). Investigate what is available locally, as well as at other universities, as there may be lectures or courses on subjects of interest to you or those you have previously not covered or thought about.

Surgery, medicine and paediatric revision courses are run by the MPS and MDU. These occur on various weekends between January and April every year. Although there are attendance fees, these are discounted if you have signed up with the defence society for your Foundation 1 year.

Finally, to maximise your learning from all these different focused experiences, the MMC Working Group for Career Management[1] suggests using a range of learning styles to help you reassess and re-evaluate your career choices and progression. You can do this by using:

- reflective logs or journal entries in learning portfolios
- debriefs of experiences in tutorials, with your educational supervisor, through appraisal, or in your peer group
- online focused experience discussions between your peers and senior colleagues
- career handbooks such as this one to help promote your reflection, so do not forget to complete the forms in Appendices 2 and 3 at each of the junctures recommended in Chapter 3.

REFERENCES

1 Modernising Medical Careers Working Group for Career Management. *Career Management: an approach for medical schools, deaneries, royal colleges and trusts.* London: Department of Health; 2005.

2 General Medical Council. *Tomorrow's Doctors.* London: General Medical Council; 1993.

3 Ciechan J, Girgis S and Smith P. *The Insiders Guide to Medical School.* 7th ed. Oxford: Blackwell Publishing; 2004.

4 www.keele.ac.uk/depts/ms/undergrad/sscs/index.htm

5 Cross P. Getting the most out of your SSMs. *StudentBMJ.* 2003; **11**: 336–7.

6 Young E, Melvin R, Coombes J, *et al.* Elect to teach. *StudentBMJ.* 2004; **12**: 36.

7 Wilson M. *The Medic's Guide to Work and Electives Around the World.* 2nd ed. Oxford: Arnold Publishers; 2004.

8 www.electives.net

9 Bong K. Buddhist medicine in occupied Tibet. *StudentBMJ.* 2004; **12**: 74–5.

10 Clompus H. Grinning in Gambia. *StudentBMJ.* 2004; **12**: 118–19.

11 Rajakumaraswamy N, Toor I and Thomas G. Transferring between medical schools. *StudentBMJ*. 2004; **12**: 20–1.

12 McManus IC, Richards P and Winder BC. Intercalated degrees, learning styles and career preferences: prospective longitudinal study of UK medical students. *BMJ*. 1999; **319**: 542–6.

13 Brown P. Research: what's the point? *StudentBMJ*. 2004; **12**: 46–7.

14 Gray LD. Erasmus: alpine retreat. *StudentBMJ*. 2003; **11**: 338.

15 Department of Health. *Operational Framework for Foundation Training. UK Foundation Programme Office*; 2007. Available at: www.foundationprogramme.nhs.uk/pages/home/key-documents (accessed 13 January 2009).

16 www.traumamedicine.org

17 www.londontraumaconference.com

18 www.rsm.ac.uk/students

19 www.pastest.co.uk

FURTHER READING

www.britishcouncil.org/erasmus

www.ifmsa.org

www.ucl.ac.uk/cihd/undergraduate

Application to Foundation Programme posts

Despite reassurance that the ratio of Foundation jobs to medical school graduates favours successful application to junior doctor jobs, this situation may change with increasing numbers of medical students. In addition, the number of jobs nationwide is irrelevant if you want to undertake your Foundation training in a specific area. The number of Foundation Programme posts is increasing year on year to accommodate the increasing number of graduates. But, because of European law, there is a potential problem because of the possible influx of European graduates applying for the Foundation Programme in the UK. Some areas also produce more medical students than there are Foundation Programme posts in their localities, which means that not all their students will be able to stay local to where they went to medical school. Competition for Foundation Programme places in these areas for students from outside medical schools will be fierce. Conversely, other areas have to actively attract students into their region for Foundation training. This chapter aims to help you with your Foundation application, from choosing rotations best suited to you to giving you guidance as to what you should be doing and when.

So, the time has come. You are facing the daunting prospect of applying for your first job as a doctor. First, some good news: in 2005 the UK had around 10% 'headroom', that is 10% more Foundation Year 1 (F1) posts than the output from medical schools;[1] even better, the BMA was quoting this figure as being around 12% in 2006. That is where the good news may be set to change. Headroom is dynamic, and with medical schools continuing to over-recruit, the BMA is concerned that previous 'headroom' figures have reduced in recent years.

The Foundation Programme is relatively new. Therefore, changes to the programme itself and to the application procedure have occurred. You will have to refer to the Foundation Programme website (www.foundationprogramme.nhs.uk) for the most up-to-date information.

HOW TO CHOOSE DEANERIES AND ROTATIONS THAT WILL SUIT YOU

Other than providing information about yourself, an important step in the application process is to apply to a Foundation school. You have to rank all UK Foundation schools in the order of your preference. Once accepted at a Foundation school (and armed with your application score) you have to rank the rotations on offer into your preferred order. Where do you start? There are a number of ways in which you can answer this question, depending on your priorities. Think about what is important to you and what you want to get from the job. Below are a number of factors that you may want to consider now and in the future when you are choosing more senior posts.

- Location of training (important for choosing your Foundation school):
  - Geographical area – do you have family commitments or dependents? Do you want to change to somewhere new or stick to where you know? Certain areas in the country have more competition for jobs than others (*see* Figure 11.1). However, beware that competition ratios can change each year.
- Type of hospital and thus experience[2] (important when choosing rotations):
  - District general hospital – may provide more experience as you will be busy and the 'patient mix' is general and representative of the normal distribution of disorders. The ratio of senior staff to junior staff is generally lower.
- Specialty interest – although you do not need to decide exactly what you want to do right now, you may want more experience in your specialty of interest or its allied specialties (*see* relevant specialty profiles in Chapter 15). If you have completed the form 'Current career interests', in Appendix 2, it would be useful to refer to it at this stage. Do not worry if you do not lean towards any particular subject as Foundation years are designed to give you a wide breadth of experience to later build on and specialise further.
- Opportunity for job satisfaction and career progression.
- Work–life balance – you can try and speak to junior doctors already in the jobs you are considering. In addition, read the flexible training section in Chapter 13.
- Money – for more information on this consult Chapter 13. Although details of banding and exact salaries are not readily available from deaneries at the application stage, you may be able to talk to current employees.
- Publishing potential – specialties such as public health often provide good opportunities for getting work published. Some consultants have a notable interest in research. You can enquire about this at the hospital or check on the relevant hospital's website.
- Confidence – it is not a good idea to rule out posts because you are not confident in the skills required. These can be practised and you will gain a lot from a rotation you are weaker in. However, it is important that you are realistic! Before you start in the position, identify any relevant weaknesses you may have so you can address them and practise specific skills if you can.

Once you have considered the above and any other personal priorities, you should research where appropriate. Try visiting the hospital, talking to staff and exploring the local area. Attempt to visualise yourself within each post, including the travelling, the nature of the work and colleagues with whom you would be working. This may help you to focus on aspects of the job not covered above. After this, take another look at the rotations on offer and see if your decision is clearer. If all this fails, Houghton[3] suggests taking notice of your gut reaction when choosing jobs!

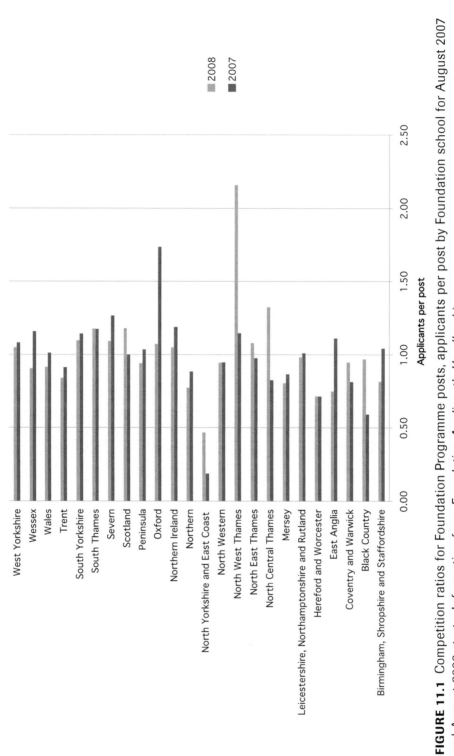

FIGURE 11.1 Competition ratios for Foundation Programme posts, applicants per post by Foundation school for August 2007 and August 2008 starts. Information from *Foundation Applicant's Handbook*[4]

APPLICATION ADVICE

The application process involves a large number of stages, which are clearly defined on the Foundation Programme website (www.foundationprogramme.nhs.uk). They will be described in brief in this section of the chapter with advice to accompany the relevant stages. However, you are strongly advised to download the current application timeline and regularly consult the Foundation Programme website for up-to-date information. The *Foundation Applicant's Handbook* available from the website is invaluable reading.[4] It provides plenty of things to do and not to do when filling out your application in addition to crib sheets and hints for answering the application questions. Do also note that the timelines and application details of the academic Foundation Programme posts are usually different and that their application deadlines are often significantly earlier. To avoid disappointment, regularly check for information of academic Foundation Posts at least six months before the usual application process opens.

The first stage in applying to the Foundation Programme is ensuring that you are, in fact, eligible to apply. This often involves no action if you are a final year student at a UK medical school; however, you may wish to chase up your medical school to ensure they have submitted the appropriate documentation to avoid disappointment. If you are applying to the Foundation Programme under different circumstances you must look at the eligibility criteria on the Foundation Programme website (www.foundationprogramme.nhs.uk) and follow the instructions regarding submission of an eligibility form and supporting documentation.[5] Make sure you investigate this early as all eligibility documentation needs to be sent together and the deadline for receiving the documents has previously been early September.

All applicants should look at the person specification, also available on the Foundation Programme website (www.foundationprogramme.nhs.uk) as this will help you to start planning the types of evidence and information you can put on your application form.

Once the application system goes live, usually in October before the August you are due to start the Foundation Programme, you can enrol onto it and download the most current version of the application form, application handbook and Foundation Programme posts. It is strongly recommended that you do this as early as possible in order to give yourself enough time to think about your answers so you may present yourself in the best way possible. Depending on your first choice Foundation school, you will be applying to either the whole two-year Foundation Programme in one go or the first year only. If the latter is true, you are usually guaranteed a job in the second year of Foundation training in the same Foundation school, although you usually have to competitively apply for the exact hospital/practice and/or rotation. Most Foundation Programme rotations consist of three four-month posts per year for two years.

You must find out the exact dates at which you can actually make your application. Give yourself plenty of time to think your answers over, but do not leave it until the very last minute before you submit your application in case of technical difficulties. Do not rely on being told the important deadlines; make sure you find them out for yourself.

The main part of your application form will consist of a series of questions, which, in total, comprise a personal statement. You must adhere to a strict word count. The exact wording of the questions varies from year to year; however the underlying principles are the same. They are usually asking you to demonstrate, through previous experiences and achievements, that you undertake constructive and effective reflective practice and that you hold the qualities of a good doctor based on the GMC document *Good Medical Practice*:[6] academic achievements, non-academic achievements, *The New Doctor* guidelines,[7] personal and education reasons for applying to first ranked Foundation school/deanery or Programme, teamwork and leadership. Check carefully that there are no spelling mistakes and computer errors – they do not look professional! Keep a copy of the form you send in, as this information may be used later, for example in an interview (if applicable).

Panels associated with the Foundation school you have applied to, will score your statements. This is done anonymously, and results in one final score that takes you through the application process. If your score does not result in a job offer from your first choice Foundation school, your documentation will be passed on to your second-ranked Foundation school and so forth until all available places have been allocated.

Your application is scored out of 100 points. A maximum of 60 points will come from your personal statement. The remaining 40 points are awarded on the basis of your academic scoring from your medical school. Your medical school is asked to submit information on where you stand in your overall academic performance compared with your year at your institution. This is done as every medical student is ranked in order of achievement and then divided into equal quartiles. You will be told by your medical school the outcome of this academic ranking.[5]

As discussed in the previous section of this chapter, your application will involve you indicating your order of preference of all the UK Foundation schools. You will also have to indicate your perceived level of competence in undertaking a given list of practical and clinical skills. The application form states that if you feel you cannot undertake any of these skills competently this information will be passed on to your future employer in order to try to give you additional support in being able to achieve them.[8]

In addition to the personal and demographic information described you will also need to provide at least two referees. It is courteous to ask permission from your referees before putting them down on your form. You must also ensure they will be available in January to March to complete your form. It is important that these referees are people with whom you have recently and closely worked. They should be consultants, GPs or associate specialists.[5] Your referees will be provided with a structured reference to complete and return once your application results have been made available and you have ranked specific programmes within your allocated Foundation school. Your references will not assist you to gain a post as they are obtained only after you have been matched to a post.

Once your references are returned and other relevant pre-employment checks have been undertaken, you will be informed of the specific programme with which you have been matched. A breakdown of your scores should be available to you and you should consider these carefully, even if you have been lucky enough to be matched with your first choice Foundation school and Programme. Try to work out what you performed well at and what you were not so good at. This will be invaluable feedback for future job applications. All that is left after this is to successfully complete your medical degree, provisionally register with the GMC and undertake further pre-employment and health checks.[8]

The following two pieces of application advice are crucial.

- Honesty is essential when applying for your Foundation jobs. A random audit of all applications is undertaken. If you make false claims you will be reported to the GMC and your career may be over before it has even started.
- If you are offered a programme you are obliged to accept this. Otherwise you can be reported to the GMC, which would jeopardise your career. Similarly if you accept a post and then change your mind and withdraw, you could be reported to the GMC.

DEVOLVED NATIONS

Applications to England, Scotland, Northern Ireland and Wales all occur initially thought the UK-wide Foundation Programme recruitment process detailed in the previous section. However, a significant addition to the application process occurs for those candidates applying to Scotland. The Scottish Foundation School covers all of Scotland, which is divided in to four deaneries: East, North, South-East and West Scotland. Once applications are received for the Scottish Foundation School through the UK-wide Foundation Programme recruitment process, the Scottish Foundation Allocation Scheme (SFAS) is undertaken. SFAS utilises a computer programme to match applicants with their programme preferences. See the SFAS website for further information (www.nes.scot.nhs.uk/sfas/)

A further consideration for Foundation Programme applicants who are moving from one country to another within the UK, is the need to be aware of the different legislation that exists. Ignorance is no defence against breaking legislation; thus you will need to brush up on law and guidance in the country you will be working in before you start.

TIMELINE FOR FOUNDATION PROGRAMME APPLICATION EVENTS

Figure 11.2 is intended as a rough guide to the timeline of events occurring as part of your Foundation Programme application. You will have to consult www. foundationprogramme.nhs.uk for accurate and up-to-date information.

SUMMARY OF GMC GUIDELINES

This section of this Handbook may trigger a groan, and that is just from those of you who have continued to read this far! However, despite the idea of reading guidelines as being time-consuming, dry and boring, it is vitally important that all medical

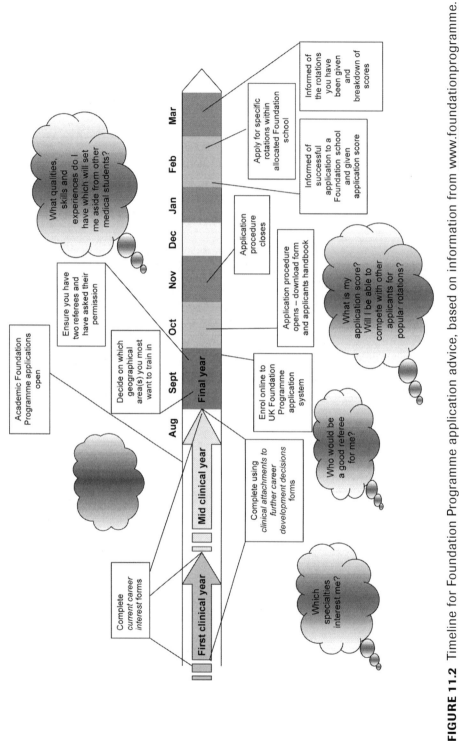

FIGURE 11.2 Timeline for Foundation Programme application advice, based on information from www.foundationprogramme.nhs.uk

students and healthcare professionals are aware of the content of the various GMC guidelines.

You are accountable to the GMC, and straying from the medical practice outlined in its guidelines will risk your professional registration and ultimately may result in you losing your job. Even as a medical student you are expected to behave and act in accordance with GMC guidance. Below are the edited highlights of the titled guidelines; by no means does this substitute for reading the guidance provided by the GMC. This section serves as an introduction and, after you have read the full guidance, it will be a source of reference to jog your memory of the content of each.

Duties of a doctor

This is fairly self-explanatory. The GMC states that the required qualities of all doctors are to:[6,9]

- make the care of your patient your *first concern*
- treat every patient *politely* and *considerately*
- respect patients' *dignity*
- give patients *information* in a way they can understand
- *respect* the rights of patients to be fully involved in decisions about their care
- keep your professional *knowledge* and *skills* up to date
- respect patients' right to *confidentiality*
- act quickly to *protect patients from risk* if you have good reason to believe that you or a colleague may be putting your patients at risk
- *protect and promote* the health of patients and the public
- support patients in *caring for themselves* to improve and maintain their health
- recognise and work within the *limits of your competence*
- *work with colleagues* in ways that best serve patients' interests
- *never discriminate unfairly* against patients or colleagues
- always be prepared to *justify your actions and decisions*.

GOOD MEDICAL PRACTICE

The *Good Medical Practice* booklet,[6] initially published in 1995 and revised in 2006, is an indexed document which expands on the duties of a doctor. It sets out guidelines, principles and standards of competent, professional care and conduct, under seven main headings.

The headings are as follows:

- Good clinical care
- Maintaining good medical practice
- Teaching and training, appraising and assessing
- Relationships with patients
- Working with colleagues
- Probity
- Health.

You should be very familiar with the guidance underlying each of these headings, not least because it outlines the behaviour expected of you as a practising doctor in the UK. At a more superficial note, the Good Medical Practice guidance is the basis of most job application forms you will have to complete in the short and intermediate term. You should therefore make sure you can link your experiences, reflective practice and activities with each of the main headings of the guidance. The GMC website (www.gmc-uk.org) is really well designed to make navigation around it easy. In addition, it provides case studies relating to each section of Good Medical Practice to enable you to understand the guidance at an even deeper level.

REFERENCES

1 Malawana J. Laying good foundations. *StudentBMJ*. 2005; **12**: 328–9.
2 Westall J. Choosing a house job. *BMJ Career Focus*. 1999; **318**: 2.
3 Houghton A. Getting that job: deciding to apply. *StudentBMJ*. 2003; **11**: 376.
4 The UK Foundation Programme Office. *FP 2009 Foundation Applicant's Handbook*. 2008. Available at: www.foundationprogramme.nhs.uk (accessed 13 January 2009).
5 Foundation Programme Office. *Foundation Programme Recruitment 2009: application process*. Available at: www.foundationprogramme.nhs.uk (accessed 13 January 2009).
6 General Medical Council. *Good Medical Practice*, 2001. Available at: www.gmc-uk.org (accessed 13 January 2009).
7 General Medical Council. *The New Doctor: recommendations on general clinical training*, 2005. Available at: www.gmc-uk.org (accessed 13 January 2009).
8 www.foundationprogramme.nhs.uk
9 General Medical Council. *The Duties of a Doctor Registered with the General Medical Council*. Available at: www.gmc-uk.org/guidance/good_medical_practice/duties_of_a_doctor.asp (accessed 8 February 2009).

FURTHER READING

British Medical Association. *Guidance on Applying for Foundation Programmes*. London: BMA; 2005.
Medical Students Committee. *Final report: BMA final year member views on application to Foundation Programmes*. London: British Medical Association; 2006.
Thomson J. Pre-registration house jobs in general practice. *BMJ Career Focus*. 1998; **317**: 2. (Good article for information on GP junior doctor jobs.)

12

The consolidation period

This chapter will provide you with an overview of what the consolidation period is and what happens during this time.

Although a 'consolidation period' may manifest itself in different ways in different medical schools, and be called a variety of names, this chapter uses the term in a generic way. The consolidation period relates to a time, usually near the end of your course, during which the main aims are to:

- round off undergraduate learning to ensure students are ready for their final exams
- facilitate the transition from medical student to junior doctor
- prepare for a lifetime of continuing learning.

The beginning of the consolidation period may be spent revising for, then sitting, your final exams. Your tutors at your university hospital(s) may provide revision sessions. However, the most help will be gained from continuing to practise clinical skills. Below, two junior doctors discuss their shadowing experience in this consolidation period.

Name: Dr Kathleen Mackie

Age: 21+ years

Position: Foundation Year 1 (F1) doctor

Hospital: University Hospital of North Staffordshire

Specialty in which shadowing took place: Vascular surgery

What shadowing involved: Basically, doing the job of a F1 doctor; that is, clerking in patients, doing simple procedures, etc.

A typical day: My experience of shadowing the F1 doctor was great. I (initially) thought four weeks was too long, especially as I had just finished my finals and wanted to start my summer holiday, but the time flew by. A typical day involved learning how my consultant likes to do things. I learnt what antibiotic regimens they liked, their anticoagulation preferences and other such useful information that made starting my job much easier. I also had to decide the order of the operating list for the next day. Other information that you learn each day whilst shadowing is which tests to order, how to get them done and how to act on their results. During the shadowing block I also met other medical students who were about to start their jobs in the same hospital. This meant that on our first day there were fewer faces that we had never seen before. As a result of completing my shadowing period I did not feel as lost or isolated as I could have done when I started my first post.

Advice for students: Good luck to you all, and enjoy your shadowing period.

Name: Dr Milan M Mehta

Age: 24 years

Position: Medical Senior House Officer

Hospital: Royal Bolton Hospital

Specialty in which shadowing occurred: PRHO medicine on gastroenterology ward

What shadowing involved: Thinking what would I do when I had to fill the shoes of the then house officer a few weeks later; for example, skills I had to learn or practise.

A typical day: 8:45 am – Help the PRHO chase up the latest blood results and mentally prepare ourselves for the consultant ward round to start shortly; 9:00 am – consultant ward round. I presented some of the patients that I clerked the day before. Whilst the PRHO presented the rest of the patients, I listed the ward round jobs; 10:30 am – the PRHO and I split the ward round jobs. I did any venflons and important blood tests that needed doing. He let me do the 'exciting' procedures (e.g. an ascitic/pleural tap or a femoral stab). I also got practice at re-writing drug charts and doing lots of discharge letters; 12 noon – lunch; 2:00 pm – second consultant ward round and, again, split the ward round jobs with the PRHO; 3:30 pm – I went home early.

Advice for students: (i) Each day ask the ward sister to tell you about the sickest patients, any new patients and then the rest of the patients, and your job will be to see the patients in that order of priority; (ii) always stay on the right side of the nurses as they have a lot of experience and will guide you through your first few weeks as a PRHO, and will often go out of their way to help you out; (iii) probably the single most important skill you need to learn as a PRHO is how to manage your time effectively.

An important aim of the final year is to facilitate the transition from being a medical student to working as a junior doctor. In the consolidation period most students have the opportunity to shadow the Foundation Year 1 Doctor (FY1) whom they will succeed in the following August. The length of this period will vary between medical schools; however, it often ranges from one week to one month. This period is included in the number of weeks of clinical training required by the GMC for provisional registration. Therefore, attendance is compulsory. Shadowing will assist students to acquire a working knowledge of their first post before taking over full responsibility for it.

At the beginning of the shadowing period most students should meet their Foundation year educational supervisor, in addition to the FY1 from whom they will be taking over. This contact with your future educational supervisor is designed to continue throughout the first post. Such early contact will provide support and allow you, as a medical student, to establish a pattern for your continuing supervision.

Different trusts and medical schools require you to undertake the consolidation period at different times. Some trainees undertake this time straight after finals in year five; others undertake the experience immediately prior to starting their FY1 jobs. If you are going to be undertaking the latter format of consolidation experience, you will be able to utilise the time by getting to know the patients on the ward, gradually taking over responsibility for their care before being left to hold the fort alone once your Foundation Programme officially starts. If your consolidation period occurs some weeks prior to the start date for your post, you can still make very good use of the time by getting to know about the systems used in the hospital. This is particularly valuable if you are going to be working in a different hospital to that in which you were a student. Find out which request forms are required for each different test, orient yourself around the hospital site and find out who all the key members of staff are. You will find that success in these activities at this stage will result in your first few days as a doctor running much more smoothly.

13

Postgraduate working conditions and pay

This chapter provides information about how your salary will be calculated, different ways you may work in the future, and advice on how to work shifts. It gives information about training schemes that help you to continue with your career under various circumstances. Finally, and, perhaps, most importantly, the chapter contains advice on how to maintain a good work–life balance.

Junior doctors' working conditions have been contentious for many years. Recently, there have been substantial changes to improve the working lives of junior doctors.

- In 2000 a new contract for junior doctors was drawn up.
- In 2001 the maximum hours worked in a week for pre-registration house officers/Foundation Year 1 doctors (PRHOs/F1s) was reduced to 56 hours.
- By 2003 all junior doctors had a maximum limit of 56 working hours per week.
- From August 2004 the European Working Time Directive (EWTD), an initiative designed to protect the health and safety of workers in the European Union, was applied to the medical profession.[1]
- By 2009 all junior doctors will work a maximum of 48 hours, averaged over a reference period.[1]

The EWTD requires that trainee doctors have 11 hours continuous rest in 24 hours; 24 hours continuous rest in 7 days (or 48 hours in 14 days); at least a 20-minute break every 6 hours; 4 weeks' annual leave and, for night workers, no more than 8 hours' work in 24 hours, averaged over a reference period.[1]

The new contract did not leave junior doctors worse off, but the EWTD has reduced their levels of pay and increased concerns about the amount of training junior doctors now receive. A positive effect of these reforms is that the working environment has been made less intense.

The salaries that junior doctors are paid relate to the hours worked and how anti-social the working hours are, as shown in Table 13.1. Based on these factors, levels of pay are organised into bands. A doctor will receive a basic salary plus a pay supplement (a percentage of the basic salary), based on the banding of that particular job.

To find out which band your posts should be awarded, visit the British Medical Association website and use their interactive banding calculators (www.bma.org.uk/employmentandcontracts/pay/basic_pay/whichband.jsp).

Your post will be monitored every six months, and you will have to fill in diary cards, as a condition of your terms and conditions of service. If your post exceeds the hours or rest requirements then you may be put into Band 3; this means you will have a multiple of 100% of your basic salary. You should then work with your trust to ensure the rota becomes legal.

If you feel your post is unfairly or incorrectly banded you can request a period of monitoring to assess the actual hours you work.

TABLE 13.1 Illustration of pay banding and supplements. For up-to-date information *see* British Medical Association website (www.bma.org.uk) or BMA *Junior Doctors' Handbook*[2]

Antisocial	Band 1: less than 48 hours/week	Band 2: 48–56 hours/week	Band 1: more than 56 hours/week
Most	50%	80%	Illegal
	Band 1A	Band 2A	
Moderate	40%	–	Illegal
	Band 1B		
Least	20%	50%	Illegal
	Band 1C	Band 2A	

A rough guide to your future pay and the increments that co-exist with career progression will now be given. However, changes in working times may result in these being incorrect in the future.

The starting annual salary for Foundation 1 (F1) doctors in August 2008 was nearly £21 000.[3] This was the basic salary before including a banding supplement. A typical new doctor in a high-intensity post would therefore receive around £30 000 per annum.[3,4] However, more and more F1 posts are totally unbanded so you should only budget on getting basic pay.

Foundation 2 (F2) doctors will earn a basic annual salary of at least £26 000.

Specialist registrars earn a basic salary of between £29 000 and £42 000, which increases to more than £60 000 per annum after supplements have been added for a typical high-intensity post.[3,4]

GP registrars receive the same basic salary as they earned in their last hospital training post. On top of this a 55% supplement is added.[3] Therefore a GP registrar who has previously been in hospital training posts for three years may earn around £46 000 per year.[3]

Consultants earn a basic salary between £67 000 and £91 000 per annum, but may receive out-of-hours supplements and clinical excellence awards. Such awards may be worth an additional £69 000, for a Platinum award, but, realistically, only very few will achieve this.[3]

Most GPs are self-employed, though some are salaried. An average full-time, self-employed GP may earn at least £72 000 per annum[4] and can earn up to £120 000 per annum.

With so many things resting on the amount you earn, it is important that you clarify exactly what your pay will be before undertaking financial commitments.

PENSIONS

All contracted NHS staff may enter the NHS pension scheme. Information on the NHS Pension Scheme in England and Wales can be found at www.nhsba.nhs.uk/pensions, information on the NHS Superannuation Scheme in Scotland can be found at www.sppa.gov.uk/nhs/home.htm, information on the Northern Ireland Health and Personal Social Services scheme can be found at www.dhsspsni.gov.uk/superann and details regarding NHS pensions can also be found on www.bma.org.uk/employmentandcontracts/pensions/index.jsp. In brief, within the scheme you will make payments amounting to 5–8.5% of your salary, to which the NHS adds the equivalent of 14% of your salary in England, Wales and Scotland and 7% in Northern Ireland. You will have the option of receiving a lump sum of money when you retire.

Changes occurred to the NHS pension schemes in March/April 2008. Make sure you research the costs and benefits of the scheme you are considering joining carefully and be careful to read the details of the new schemes if you have not joined them before this change.

The BMA website (www.bma.org.uk/employmentandcontracts/pensions/pension_scheme./index.jsp) contains lots of useful information regarding pensions and contains downloadable fact sheets for various specific circumstances that might affect your pension. Situations covered include voluntary early retirement, maternity/paternity leave, redundancy and working abroad. Make sure you look into the implications on your pension should you choose to spend some time working abroad. The BMA's *Junior Doctors' Handbook* warns you that if you have been working for less than two years and are away from the NHS for more than a year then a refund of contributions is normally payable. The *Handbook* highlights the negative result this has as your repayment will be reduced through taxation and payment of national insurance contributions.[2]

PRIVATE PRACTICE

The NHS was founded in 1948 to provide healthcare, free at the point of use. Since the creation of the NHS, the private sector has become relatively small, with only 11% of the population having private healthcare insurance.[5]

For GPs there is no limit on receiving income through private practice and commercial contracts, provided NHS commitments are met.[5] However, if NHS premises are used, and more than 10% of the money earned by the practice is through non-NHS work, the primary care trust will proportionally reduce the reimbursements to the practice.[4]

Consultants have no restriction on their private earnings under the new consultant contract.[5] They must only demonstrate that they are fulfilling their NHS job plan, and there must be no conflict of interest between NHS work and private practice work.[5] For junior doctors and staff-grade doctors there is also no limit on private practice provided that the private work is done outside contracted hours and does not interfere with their duties.[5]

Your trust, who is your main employer, is entitled to know of any work you carry out outside your normal contracted hours. It is entitled to prohibit you from other employment if it is felt that this interferes with the service you give to the trust. Trusts are also entitled to know if you are doing extra locums; you may be prohibited from doing these if they interfere with your training, or trust service. Private hospitals will not give admitting rights to anyone but those on the Specialist Register. Your NHS indemnity will not cover any other form of private activity so you will need to arrange additional, private indemnity insurance.

Junior doctors, including GP registrars, should seek the agreement of the relevant consultant or GP trainer, before doing any private practice.[5] Realistically, permission would rarely be granted as extra work is likely to impinge on doctors' capacity to learn and develop in their training posts.

A controversial issue with private practice is the perceived 'queue jumping' by private patients. The truth is that British patients may opt into or out of NHS-funded treatment at any stage.[5] However, patients who have had a private consultation initially, but then re-enter NHS-funded treatment, should be placed at the same position on the waiting list as if their original consultation had been within the NHS.[5] Although the GMC allows doctors to advertise their services publicly, it is unethical to spend time discussing or promoting private practice during NHS consultations.[5]

LOCUM WORK

Locum doctors are 'stand-in' doctors, who cover the work of permanent doctors who are sick, on annual leave or away from work for any other reason. Locums can also be appointed to cover a position that has not yet been filled. You can only work as a locum if you are qualified to the degree that is required by the position you are 'stepping into'. You must also be covered by appropriate indemnity insurance. If you have a full-time NHS post, your trust is entitled to know if you are doing extra locum sessions.

To work as a locum doctor in hospital or general practice, you may wish to register with a locum agency or you can be employed directly; remuneration from each source of work may be different, and you will have to investigate this to get the best deal. You can register with as many agencies as you wish and you have no commitments until you accept a locum position. The positive points about locum work are that you:

- know how much and how often you will receive your money once the work is arranged
- can work flexibly (i.e. not tied down to a contract)
- can work in the location you desire
- can earn money whilst planning a career change, travel, etc.

The negative points about locum work include:

- an unpredictable income
- no paid study leave or annual leave
- no chance to familiarise yourself with a hospital

- it usually does not count towards training
- having to become familiar with the requirements of being self-employed (e.g. income tax, National Insurance, keeping accounts) if you are working in general practice (unless you are employed by an agency).

To work as a GP locum you need to be on an NHS trust performers' list.

SHIFT WORK

Working horrendous shifts was once seen as a rite of passage into the upper ranks of the medical profession. Doctors used to work a normal day and then remain on-call through the night or weekend.[6] This caused disruption to their circadian rhythms, resulting in daytime sleepiness and fatigue.

Rotational shifts are a good way of organising shift work. The best rotating shift is the fast-forward rotation.[6] An example of this shift pattern is to work two mornings then two afternoons and then two nights. The worst shift pattern is the opposite, the backward-rotating shift. This would involve, for example, a week of nights then a week of afternoons then a week of mornings.

Shift work, especially at night, has many negative effects on junior doctors, which include:[6]

- disruption of the normal circadian rhythm
- 'shift lag' – short-term sleepiness, insomnia, digestive problems and reduced mental agility
- significant effects on performance – studies of practical ability and efficiency show significant dips occur between 10:00 pm and 6:00 am, with a trough at 3:00 am[6]
- sleep disturbance
- loss of rapid eye movement during sleep.

The physical risks of shift work include:[6]

- peptic ulcer disease
- coronary heart disease
- miscarriage, low birth weight and pre-term birth
- injury (which is more likely to occur during night shifts compared to day shifts).

The risks and effects of shift work illustrate the importance of learning how to protect your health while working shifts, especially night shifts. Here are a few tips to help you when you are working night shifts:[6]

- take short breaks every hour
- only drink coffee in the first half of the shift
- take a main meal break between midnight and 1:00 am – eat a protein-rich or health food
- take a smaller food break between 3:00 am and 4:00 am
- take naps to reduce sleepiness, but be aware of sleep inertia: a period of reduced

alertness 5–15 minutes after waking
● avoid driving to or from work
● eat healthily and stay fit
● avoid shift work if you are pregnant.

Sleep disturbance is the most common effect of shift work. Tips to deal with this include:[6]
● ensure the room you sleep in is quiet and darkened
● avoid caffeine, smoking, alcohol and sleeping pills
● some people find taking melatonin before trying to sleep helps (consult appropriately trained health professionals before trying this).

The EWTD requires employers to assess the health of shift workers free of charge and at regular intervals. This is usually done using a questionnaire that is completed every three years for those under the age of 45 years and every two years for those over the age of 45 years.

FLEXIBLE WORKING

Flexible training scheme

The flexible training scheme allows doctors to work 'less than full-time' in posts that are fully recognised for training and have the educational approval of the Postgraduate Medical Education and Training Board (PMETB) by recommendation of the postgraduate deaneries and royal colleges.[7] Flexible training posts are available for doctors who are unable to train full-time for good reasons.

More recent arrangements allow flexible training to be undertaken for other reasons such as specific religious roles, training for significant sporting events or holding short-term posts with 'extraordinary responsibility'.[2] There is a significant call for flexible training. The *National Survey of Trainees 2007*, undertaken by the PMETB, reports that 22% of women and 7% of men wish to train flexibly, but currently are not doing so. The proportion of flexible trainees was also found to vary by specialty, with the surgical specialties having the fewest flexible trainees.[8] Therefore, if you want to be a flexible trainee, make sure you actively pursue it so you do not become one of these statistics.

There are four types of flexible training placements.[7]

1 Flexible/supernumerary posts – additional to the normal complement of trainees in a particular specialty.
2 Part-time, working reduced hours in a full-time slot (applies mainly to specialist registrars) – a trainee reduces the hours they work, for example having a full weekday off, working half-days or having flexible start and finish times.
3 Slot share – two flexible trainees cover the duties of a full-time post. Each post should include between 50% and 70% of full-time hours and last for 6 or 12 months. Slot share partners may change depending on individual training needs.
4 Job-share – a training placement is divided between two trainees. The two trainees cover all the original duties of a full-time post. No eligibility criteria is

required if the employer is satisfied that the job-sharers are the best candidates at appointment. The two candidates must send in a joint application, plan how to work together to obey their contractual obligations and decide how they will divide annual/study leave and pay.

The associate dean for flexible training decides at a confidential meeting whether or not a candidate's reasons are well founded and thus whether or not they receive the flexible training post.[7]

If you are interested in joining a flexible training scheme you can find out more information from your (prospective) deanery's website. Each deanery will have a designated associate dean with responsibility for flexible training and you may wish to contact them with specific questions. Once you have made your decision to apply for flexible training let your deanery know at the earliest possible time and follow the application instructions found on their website. Information for those who wish to undertake flexible Specialty Training can be found in *The Gold Guide* available from the MMC website (www.mmc.nhs.uk).[9]

Flexible Careers Scheme

The Flexible Careers Scheme[10] allows consultants, GPs and hospital doctors of all grades to work up to 50% of full-time. The scheme was developed to provide doctors with an opportunity to work flexibly whilst being supported in maintaining their career. The range of doctors who use this scheme include those who want to work less than 50% of full-time, those who are, or will soon be, retired and those who want to return to work in medicine but need a period of supervised work.

Until 2005, NHS professionals were responsible for the Flexible Careers Scheme, working in partnership with local postgraduate deaneries in England.[10] The scheme could be adapted to suit individual needs and provided enough clinical practice for revalidation purposes.[10] There was a limit to how long a person could stay on the Flexible Careers Scheme, but extensions were possible.[10] At the end of 2005, the funding for the scheme was devolved by the Department of Health to local NHS organisations. If you are interested in joining the Flexible Careers Scheme contact your employer to find out if and how it is run in your area.[7]

WORK–LIFE BALANCE

Research has shown that there are three types of hospital consultant in terms of work–life balance. These types are described based on the relation between their career and their personal or family lives.[11]

- Career-dominant:
  - characteristics: single, divorced, childless
  - career course: full-time, continuous
  - reflections: female – some made a conscious decision not to have a family; both males and females – some expressed strong regrets about neglecting their lives outside medicine.
- Segregated:

- characteristics: married/divorced, with/without children, family responsibilities organised to enable more time to be involved in their career
- career course: full-time, continuous
- reflections: male – many dissatisfied with their work–life balance and blame pressure to conform to intensive work practices; female – many believed this approach was the only way to achieve consultant grades and have a family.
- Accommodating:
  - characteristics: married/cohabiting, children
  - career course: males – full-time, continuous; females – career break and/or periods of part-time training/work
  - reflections: both males and females expressed satisfaction with their work–life balance.[11]

In order for you to achieve your perfect balance of working towards and within a career in medicine, and living a life outside medicine, you must think about:[12]
- your own definition of happiness
- your perfect day in the future
- how you will get to your perfect life.

You must also think about how you will cope with the risks to your standard of living that come with a career in medicine, for example:[13]
- high prevalence of stress
- discordance between public image and realities of your job
- low morale
- high divorce rate
- high risk of substance and alcohol abuse.

A tip to assist you with contemplating your ideal work–life balance is to devise a life strategy with goals. You should think about the path to reach your goals as well as any obstacles you may face both in your work and personal lives.[13]

When you are working as a doctor, managing your work–life balance will initially involve thinking about the purpose of your life and its importance to others. You should reflect on your current work–life balance and what areas of your life you may be neglecting.[14] A good way of doing this is to list eight roles that you occupy (including your role as your own body's carer), and then rate how well you fulfil those roles on a scale of 1 to 10.[14] Not only will this provide you with an overview of your life, but also you will easily see if you are neglecting any role.[14] You can then direct your energy towards the roles that require increased attention and improved performance.

In order to be happy whilst working in medicine it is important to remain fit and spend enough time concentrating on non-medical things. You should deal promptly with any problems as they arise. Problems can occur in many areas of your non-medical life, and you should monitor your health, finances, relationships and social life, in order to pick up difficulties early on.[13]

Help with managing your work–life balance is available from the Royal Medical

Benevolent Fund (RMBF). The RMBF website (www.support4doctors.org) is an independent and non-judgemental source of support that includes:

- information on how to find different sources of support (e.g. information on careers, finance, health and family life)
- contact details for peer support telephone helplines
- information on achieving a good work–life balance.

REFERENCES

1 Department of Health. *Guidance on Working Patterns for Junior Doctors*, 2002. Available at: www.dh.gov.uk/prod_consum_dh/groups/dh_digitalassets/@dh/@en/documents/digitalasset/dh_4069967.pdf (accessed 8 February 2009).

2 British Medical Association Junior Doctors Committee. *Junior Doctors' Handbook*. London: British Medical Association; 2008.

3 British Medical Association. *Guidance Note Supplement. Doctors' pay: current levels*. British Medical Association. Last revision December 2008. Available at: www.bma.org.uk/images/docspaysuppl_tcm41-147308.pdf (accessed 14 January 2009).

4 British Medical Association. *Fees for Part-time Medical Service*; 2004. Available at: www.bma.org.uk/employmentandcontracts/independent_medical_practice/focusprivatepractice0604.jsp#Appendix1 (accessed 8 February 2009).

5 British Medical Association. *A Code of Practice for Private Practice*; 2004. Available at: www.bma.org.uk/employmentandcontracts/independent_medical_practice/CCSCContractprivMS.jsp (accessed 8 February 2009).

6 Hobson J. Shift work and doctors' health. *BMJ Career Focus*. 2004; **329**: 149–50.

7 West Midlands Deanery. *Flexible Careers and Training*. Available at: www.wmdeanery.org/careerguide/flextraining.asp (accessed 14 January 2009).

8 Postgraduate Medical Education and Training Board. *National Survey of Trainees 2007 Summary Report*. Postgraduate Medical Education and Training Board: London. Available at: www.pmetb.org.uk/fileadmin/user/QA/Trainee_Survey/National_Survey_of_Trainees_2007_Summary_Report_20080723-Final.pdf (accessed 14 January 2009).

9 Department of Health. *A Reference Guide for Postgraduate Specialty Training in the UK*. 2nd ed. London: Department of Health; 2008. Available at: www.mmc.nhs.uk/default.aspx?page=457 (accessed 8 February 2009).

10 Department of Health. *Flexible Working for Doctors Highlighted*, 2003. Available at: www.dh.gov.uk/en/Publicationsandstatistics/Pressreleases/DH_4047391 (accessed 14 January 2009).

11 Dumelow C, Littlejohns P and Griffiths S. Relation between a career and family for English hospital consultants: qualitative semi-structured interview study. *BMJ*. 2000; **320**: 1437–40.

12 Steel N. Planning your life and career. *BMJ Career Focus*. 1999; **319**: 2.

13 Gray C. Life, your career and the pursuit of happiness. *BMJ Careers*. 1997; **315**: 2.

14 Houghton A. Personal support 3: how to help someone achieve balance in their working and personal lives. *BMJ Career Focus*. 2005; **331**: 7–8.

FURTHER READING

BMA website (www.bma.org.uk).

14

Specialty training

The specialty and general practice training programme is competitive – just as it is for Foundation Programme posts (*see* Chapter 9).[1] Among other things, the selection process utilises information and experience gathered during your Foundation Programme. This chapter will describe the specialty and GP training structure as correct at the time of printing, highlight the areas that may change and give you general advice on how to apply for a specialty or GP training post.

Application and selection onto these higher training programmes currently occurs prior to the end of your Foundation training. Therefore it is crucial that during medical school and your Foundation training you are thinking hard about what specialties you may be interested in and, if not, those you definitely are not considering undertaking long term. In addition to the tools described in Chapter 3 and speaking with your educational/clinical supervisor(s) and perhaps a mentor, the specialty profiles found in Chapter 15 will provide you with a basic overview of each of the main specialties. Further information regarding each specialty can be sought in the career section of West Midlands Workforce Deanery website (www. westmidlands.nhs.uk/WorkforceDeanery/MedicalCareers/tabid/68/Default.aspx) which contains not only written information but podcasts about a large number of specialties. The Modernising Medical Careers (MMC) initiative promoted career support throughout medical school and your Foundation training. Therefore, you should be able to get help locally in making career decisions. The BMA has published a document, *Medical Specialties: the way forward*,[2] that contains a section on choosing the correct specialty for you, information about the different specialty options (including specialty profiles) and other options that are also available, such as armed forces, private practice, medical journalism and working abroad. This is well worth a read.

There have been multiple changes to the specialty application procedures over recent years as described in Chapter 8. At the time of printing further changes are yet to be announced for the next round of applications. However, whatever the specific structure of the application system, general principles remain consistent. Therefore, the rest of this chapter will give you both generic and specific information on specialty and GP application processes in more detail. Don't forget that specific information regarding individual specialties, training schemes and application advice can be found on the relevant royal college web pages (*see* Appendix 6) as well as deanery web pages.

GUIDANCE ABOUT SPECIALTY TRAINING

The Gold Guide has been published by the Department of Health on the MMC website, which is *A Reference Guide for Postgraduate Specialty Training in the UK*. At the time of print the second edition was the most current and applied to all specialty trainees who commenced Specialty Training on or after 6th August 2008.[3] *The Gold Guide* outlines the statutory bodies, characteristics of Specialty Training, standards that apply to Specialty Training programmes and becoming and progressing as a specialty registrar.

Every junior trainee should look through the most current version of *The Gold Guide* – it is essential reading.

GAINING EXPERIENCE PRIOR TO APPLICATION

Contrary to some beliefs, you do not have to have done a Foundation post in the exact field in which you want to specialise. However, it is expected that you have gained some experience in related or relevant areas. The specialty profiles found in Chapter 15 should assist you in finding allied areas in which to gain experience. In addition, don't forget about taster experiences, which are available to Foundation trainees. These allow you to spend one or two weeks away from your usual clinical post shadowing doctors in a specialty you are considering (*see* Chapter 10 for more information).

Audits are a means by which you can find out more about a specific topic, improve clinical performance and improve your CV. If you have an interest in a particular specialty, you could make links with local colleagues in that specialty in order to undertake an audit.

Application help, guidance and support can be gained from senior colleagues as well as professional organisations. For example, information gain be obtained from BMJ Careers (http://careers.bmj.com), BMJ Career Fairs (http://careersfair.bmj.com) and Medical Forum (www.medicalforum.com).

WHAT ARE YOU APPLYING TO?

The current situation is that for some specialties, run-through training is available (i.e. once you have been appointed a post you remain in this training scheme until awarded your Certificate of Completion of Training [CCT] provided you satisfactorily meet all requirements) and in others, specialties are uncoupled (i.e. you first apply to a broad based core Specialty Training programme before competitively applying to Specialty Training posts with a narrower specialty theme that leads you to your CCT). However, if the Tooke recommendations are implemented, it is likely more postgraduate pathways will follow the structure of the present uncoupled jobs. It is important that you know exactly what you are applying for as you may need to prepare for competitive job applications within two to three years after securing your first post in an uncoupled specialty. Other, non-training, jobs are also available so do make sure you are not confused about the future prospects of the post you are applying to.

PREPARING FOR APPLICATION

From 2008, applications into Specialty Training have generally been deanery led, which followed on from well-publicised problems with a centrally organised recruitment system 'MTAS' (Medical Training Application System). However, a few specialties continue to have central application systems because either they have successfully established central recruitment systems and/or they are relatively small. For example, applications to all levels of general practice, histopathology, obstetrics and gynaecology, public health and paediatrics and applications to Specialty Training Year 3 in cardiothoracic surgery, neurosurgery and plastic surgery.[4] Jobs are therefore advertised on individual deanery websites, but they can also be found in the BMJ, on BMJ Careers website (http://careers.bmj.com/careers/welcome.html) and on the NHS Jobs website (www.jobs.nhs.uk). Academic Specialty Training jobs can be found on the National Institute for Health Research (NIHR) Coordinating Centre for Research Capacity Development website (www.nccrcd.nhs.uk).

Local recruitment processes may not be enduring; however, lessons have been learnt from 2007 and if a national recruitment process is to be reintroduced in the future it will have to first undergo rigorous piloting. Therefore, local recruitment is likely to continue at least in the short-term.

Think about how competitive your application is likely to be. Although the overall competition ratio is about three doctors to every one post, this ratio alters by specialty and geographical area. For example, jobs in London are usually very oversubscribed.[5]

A paper in BMJ Careers by West and Douglas that described experiences of surgical training applications in 2007–08 stated the following information was required on most or all of the application forms:[6]

- audit work – including an understanding of the audit process
- experience and participation in research – often only when work has been accepted/published in peer reviewed journals
- exams passed – dates and sometimes number of attempts
- courses – make sure you try to attend all core specialty specific courses on offer (e.g. Advanced Trauma Life Support if you are applying to emergency medicine)
- clinical (and where relevant, operative) experience – this may take the form of a logbook, having to state the number of times you have performed particular procedures or reflection on particular clinical encounters. Therefore, when applicable, make sure you keep your log books up to date
- commitment to the specialty – you must demonstrate why you want the job in that particular specialty and the lengths you have gone to in order to prepare for a career in this specialty.

For further information about what to include in some of these headings and also further headings that may be covered in an application form can be found in Chapter 4 under advice about CVs. You should spend time in the period leading up to Specialty Training applications making your CV as comprehensive as possible and frequently reflecting on your clinical experiences, both good and bad, in order to make completion of applications as easy as possible.

There is great concern among junior doctors about securing higher training posts, especially following the recruitment problems resulting from a national application process in 2007. To maximise your chances of securing a higher training post you must be flexible about the geographical area and/or specialty(ies) to which you apply. This is fine if you are most concerned about job security; however, if you are dead set about working in a certain specialty and none other will suffice, you will have to first ensure that your CV, and subsequent application, is top notch, but you should also strongly consider 'back-up options'.

Specialty Training applications generally open in early January and close in May; however this may be subject to change and you are strongly advised to keep checking for application timetables on the deanery websites from at least three months prior to these dates to ensure you give yourself plenty of time to prepare. Some deaneries request that you register prior to undertaking the application process. Applications for academic clinical fellowships for the integrated clinical and academic posts usually open earlier than the main round. Often the applications open and close in November ready for interviews in January. Previously, applications for GP academic programmes have occurred at the same time as the main recruitment process, but do check this if you are interested. There has been a suggestion to introduce multiple recruitment rounds throughout the year to prevent mass changeover of doctors. This requires further planning before implementation as all Foundation trainees reach their end point at the same time. Just be aware that this has potential to change over forthcoming years.[7]

SUBMITTING YOUR APPLICATION

During the time period when applications are 'live' you must be on the ball and regularly checking jobs. They may only be advertised for 72 hours and you would not want to miss out on your dream job because you are not checking for posts regularly enough. Once a job has been advertised you will have at least 5 days to apply electronically; this timeframe increases to 10 days if you have to send in a paper application. Ensure you have the current contact details of and permission from your previous three clinical/educational supervisors so you avoid delays in completing your application.

If you are applying to specialties without central application systems be prepared to complete a number of application forms in a very short space of time. For most specialties, each individual deanery will create their own application and scoring systems. Usually application forms are structured and contain various quantities of CV-based material 'white-box' questions (i.e. questions for which you have to provide a short paragraph as an answer, much like a personal statement) and specialty-specific questions. Don't get too hung up on knowing exactly what the form will look like. You may end up completing different multiple forms. Instead, think more about how you will approach answering the questions. You will now be grateful you have kept your CV up to date and if you haven't, now is the time to do so. Before you start, ensure you have entered all your information on to a master CV. Even if you don't need to include the full CV, having all your skills, achievements and qualifications laid out in one document makes it a lot easier to complete white box questions. In addition, ensure your reflective practice diary, portfolio and/or skills log are contemporary and full as many questions asked on the application form can be answered directly from these records if they are of high quality.

Ensure you answer the questions asked of you as fully as you can. Even if you think the only evidence you have for a certain attribute is soft, it is better than no evidence at all.[8] Make full use of your word count, but cut out all words that do not add to your answer to make your answer rich, sharp and succinct. For every answer you write, you must be willing to speak about it in full and it must be entirely truthful.

Carefully read the person specifications and eligibility for the jobs you are applying for. Not only do you want to check you are not wasting your (and the shortlisters') time, but also you should use the person specification to mould your answers on the application form to ensure you fully demonstrate your suitability to the job.

Do not wait until the last moment to complete and submit your application. Ensure you leave time to check your answers through carefully, typos and poor grammar can lead to your otherwise strong application being rejected. Avoid acronyms as they can cause confusion. Beware of additional pages or forms that require completion and submission with your application.[8] Make sure you have read everything at least a couple of times and get at least one colleague you trust to read it through also to make sure you haven't missed anything and that your answers fully answer the questions asked of you. Also allow for any technical problems, for example, computers can crash, internet service can be interrupted and postal workers can go on strike. Don't let any of these problems stop your application reaching its destination on time.

Print and save a hard copy of your application. You will need this to help you prepare for your interview if your application is successful.

WHAT HAPPENS NEXT?

First make sure your application has definitely arrived, having sent it is not synonymous with the correct people having received it.[8] Depending on the deanery and specialty, what happens after you submit your application form will be different. However one thing that is consistent is that all applications are scored and applicants with the highest scores will be shortlisted. Usually, if you are shortlisted you will be invited to an interview process. This may range through anything from a panel interview to an examination and selection day. For example, applicants to the GP training scheme are invited to undertake written exams as part of the short-listing process. Those who are shortlisted are then invited to the selection day in which a group activity, a communication station and another written exercise are undertaken. You may wish to study for these exams and for the activities on the selection day well in advance so make sure you find out about the entire application process before it is underway. Recommendations for wide use of exams within selection processes have been made, so look out for this change being implemented.[7] For more information on interviews *see* Chapter 4.

If you are lucky enough to be offered a job you must be sure you want it before accepting it. If you accept a job then later turn it down you may be liable to being reported to the GMC. Prior to starting your new job you will have to undergo a police check, occupational health review and GMC validation check.

Your deanery should issue you with a national training number (NTN) within a month of you starting your Specialty Training, provided you have accepted the *Conditions of Taking up a Training Post*. The NTN is essential as it ensures your Annual Review of Competence Progression is initiated and it results in your postgraduate dean forwarding a copy of your registration to the relevant royal college or faculty. It also records your date of entry on to the programme. To find this and further information on the NTN read *The Gold Guide*.[3]

Specific details on the work-based assessments, records of clinical skills, portfolios, appraisals, Annual Review of Competence Progression and exam requirements differ for every specialty. However, it is crucial that you are familiar with what is required from you right from the start as on-call shifts, annual leave, study leave and other commitments result in the time flying past quickly and it is easy to get behind. General information is found in *The Gold Guide*;[3] however, for specialty-specific information visit the appropriate royal college and/or faculty website. Also speak with your educational supervisor early to plan how you will achieve all that is required of you.

UNDERTAKING SPECIALTY TRAINING

You will undertake your Specialty Training under the guidance of an educational supervisor, much like that during the Foundation Programme. It is essential that you make early contact with your educational supervisors and that you record all meetings you have with them in your portfolio (*see* below). It is through discussion with your educational supervisor and with reference to your curriculum that you will be able to set learning needs, create your personal development plan and gauge your progress towards your final goal of a CCT.

Current Specialty Training curricula are approved by the PMETB. The PMETB have written *Generic Standards for Training*, which are available for free download from their website, to which Specialty Training curricular and standards should meet.[9] The curricula for each specialty can be found on the appropriate royal college and/or faculty website.

To successfully complete Specialty Training and to obtain a CCT, you must undertake the required assessments, appraisals and an annual review. If you are in a surgical specialty, for example, you may also be required to undertake a number of specific procedures. All of your educational, training and personal development activities are collated within your portfolio and/or logbook. Increasingly, portfolios and logbooks have become electronic, accessed online through the relevant royal college and/or faculty websites. It is essential that you collate your portfolio/logbook, however to obtain a password you have to register with the royal college/faculty and often pay a reasonable sum of money. Once you have access to your portfolio/logbook you must keep it contemporary and well maintained. Your portfolio and/or logbook are the only sources of objective evidence of your progress as well as evidence that you are a self-sufficient learner and that you are working towards achieving your set learning needs.

At some stage during your Specialty Training you will have to undertake post-graduate exams, often these are membership exams for the royal college relevant to your specialty. The timing of these exams varies for each specialty and between trainees within specialties. You should access the appropriate royal college website, ideally prior to applying to your Specialty Training posts, but if you have missed this chance, find out as soon as possible when you are expected to undertake the exams, what they involve and how many you will have to take. Some exam results can only be held for a fixed time period before you receive your CCT, so make sure that you do not take them too early.

INTER-DEANERY TRANSFERS

Moving from one deanery to another once your Specialty Training is underway is possible. However, a transfer must occur for well-founded personal reasons and must not confer an advantage to you; that is, you cannot move from an uncoupled to a coupled training post without going through the usual competitive recruitment process. Details of the inter-deanery transfer process, eligible and ineligible reasons for wanting to transfer and what to do if your request is not supported, are given in *The Gold Guide*.[3]

SPECIALTY TRAINING IN DEVOLVED NATIONS

Although the general principles are the same, much of the above information relates to the Specialty Training applications in England. For country-specific information on Specialty Training and applications make sure you visit the appropriate sites:

- MMC England website Specialty Training information can be found at www. mmc.nhs.uk/default.aspx?page=315
- MMC Scotland Specialty Training information can be found at www.mmc.scot. nhs.uk
- MMC in Wales Specialty Training information can be found at www. mmcwales.org/specialty-training
- Northern Ireland Medical and Dental Training Agency Specialty Training information can be found at www.nimdta.gov.uk/hospital-medicine/specialties/

REFERENCES

1 Department of Health. *Modernising Medical Careers: the next steps.* 2004. Available at: www. dh.gov.uk/en/Publicationsandstatistics/Publications/PolicyAndGuidance/DH_4079530 (accessed 8 February 2009).
2 British Medical Association Medical Education Sub-committee of the Board of Science. *Medical Specialties: the way forward.* London: British Medical Association; 2007.
3 Department of Health. *A Reference Guide for Postgraduate Specialty Training in the UK.* 2nd ed. London: Department of Health; 2008. Available at: www.mmc.nhs.uk/default.aspx?page=457 (accessed 8 February 2009).

4 Modernising Medical Careers. *Training FAQs.* Available at: www.mmc.nhs.uk/default.aspx? page=320 (accessed 14 January 2009).

5 www.mmc.nhs.uk

6 West CC, Douglas H. *A Guide to Completing Core Surgical Training Application Forms: experiences from 2007 and 2008.* BMJ Careers; 2008. Available at: http://careers.bmj.com/careers/advice/view-article.html?id=3016 (accessed 14 January 2009).

7 Secretary of State for Health. *The Government Response to the Health Select Committee Report 'Modernising Medical Careers'.* Norwich: The Stationery Office; 2008.

8 Cater S. *How to Fill in an Application Form for a Specialist Post.* BMJ Careers; 2008. Available at: http://careers.bmj.com/careers/advice/view-article.html?id=2842 (accessed 14 January 2009).

9 Postgraduate Medical Education and Training Board. *Generic Standards for Training.* London: Postgraduate Medical Education and Training Board; 2007.

FURTHER READING

British Medical Association Medical Education Sub-committee of the Board of Science. *Medical Specialties: the way forward.* London: British Medical Association; 2007.

Specialty profiles

15

Within this chapter you will find a number of specialty profiles. These have been created by professionals who work in each of the different specialties. Whether or not you know what you want to do with your career, these may provide you with vital information.

When choosing a specialty that you will apply to work in long term, it is really important that you know not only what it involves but also what skills are required and what the downsides are. You need to match all of this information with reflection about your own desires, skills and likes/dislikes to ensure you make the right decision for you. Included in this chapter are a large number of specialty profiles. We do not expect you to read them all, but to dip in and out of those that interest you and/or that you have not heard much about.

If you like a more interactive style of information delivery, visit the career section of the West Midlands Workforce Deanery website (http://workforcedeanery. westmidlands.nhs.uk/Medicalanddental/ACareerinMedicine/Podcasts/tabid/175/ Default.aspx) to access a number of pod-casts describing careers in different specialties.

For up-to-date information on training length, visit the appropriate royal college website (found at the bottom of each specialty profile). Competition ratios for each specialty can be found at the time of printing on the Modernising Medical Careers website (www.mmc.nhs.uk). However, be warned that competition ratios for specialties can vary from year to year.

Specialty profile: A&E

Name: Dr Arvinder Sadana

Position: Consultant in Emergency Medicine (A&E)

Hospital: St George's, London

Daily activities: Vary enormously, but supervision of junior staff is the most important and enjoyable part. Teaching, administration and meetings comprise most of the time. Typically, I start work between 8:00 am and 8:30 am, attend an escalation meeting for 10–15 minutes, assess the 'state' of the department, perform 'shop floor' work or do administration or teaching, etc. I usually leave at around 6:00 pm.

Qualities required: Ability to 'multi-task', flexibility/adaptability, sense of humour, ability to stay calm at all (well, most) times.

Pros: Interesting, challenging and unpredictable work; a lot of flexibility; good team spirit.

Cons: These change, but currently pressures imposed by central government to meet targets seem to override other priorities.

Sub-specialties: Recognised sub-specialties in the UK are paediatrics and intensive care. Most A&E consultants will have their own particular interests; mine are toxicology, acute medicine and observation wards.

Allied specialties: Most other specialties are useful, but in particular, general medicine, cardiology, anaesthetics/ITU, paediatrics, orthopaedics and some general surgery.

Royal college website address: www.rcplondon.ac.uk

Specialty profile: Acute Medicine

Name: Dr Tunku Muzafar Shah

Position: Consultant in Acute Medicine

Hospital: University Hospital of Wales, Cardiff and Vale

Daily activities: Assess patient status in the medical assessment unit; review and optimise management of newly admitted and acutely ill patients; run review and follow-up clinics. In addition there may be other professional activities, sub-specialty sessions, teaching, audit, research and organisational activities (the specialty is relatively new).

Qualities required: Affinity towards medicine and the variety it can offer; must enjoy dealing with acutely ill patients; good leadership skills; team player; decisive.

Allied specialties: Cardiology; diabetes and endocrinology; gastroenterology; geriatrics and care of the elderly; medical assessment/admissions unit; intensive care; nephrology; respiratory.

Royal college website address: www.rcplondon.ac.uk

Specialty profile: Age-Related Medicine

Name: Dr A Y Chaudhry

Position: Consultant Physician in Acute Medicine and Gerontology Department

Hospital: University Hospitals Coventry and Warwickshire NHS Trust

Daily activities: Ward round for inpatients three times per week, outpatients clinics and multi-disciplinary team meetings, teaching, academic meetings and meeting with relatives.

Qualities required: Good time-management skills are essential. An understanding of what the job entails, as it can be frustrating when you are very busy and your contemporaries are having time free. Good communication skills, particularly with relatives.

Pros: Excellent opportunity to learn acute medicine along with basic practical procedures; good team spirit; opportunities for involvement in audit and academic activities; excellent opportunity for holistic approach to patient care.

Cons: Very busy job; frustrating delayed discharges due to community social issues.

Sub-specialties: Falls; transient ischaemic attacks; stroke; rehabilitation; Parkinson's disease.

Allied specialties: Orthogeriatric; geriatric psychiatry; palliative care. Students would be advised to consider part-time work (e.g. as a healthcare assistant) in this specialty if you have not had previous exposure.

Royal college website address: www.rcplondon.ac.uk; British Geriatric Society (www.bgs.org.uk).

Specialty profile: Anaesthetics

Name: Dr Keith Clayton

Position: Consultant Anaesthetist, Honorary Senior Lecturer University of Warwick; Chair, Hospital Transfusion Committee

Hospital: University Hospitals Coventry and Warwickshire NHS Trust, Warwick

Daily activities: I usually arrive at C&W at about 7:50 am to see patients and set up for an early start. I aim to finish at about 5:00 pm with no lunch break. In an average week I will also lecture at the medical school. Throughout the week I work in theatre on a variety of cases, including ophthalmology, breast surgery and orthopaedics. I also work with patients requiring pain relief.

Qualities required: Knowledgeable; team player; good communicator; dextrous; extrovert. Leadership qualities develop over the years.

Pros: Our on-call commitment on the general rota is about 1 in 20, which is extremely civilised. You pick on-call days which are convenient to you, for example four Mondays and a weekend. You get to work in teams that develop over the years. You can change your sessions over the years – I did 10 years of obstetric anaesthesia before changing my sessions around. It gives you the ability to have a new job every few years. There are opportunities to work in ITU, chronic pain, acute pain, neuro, cardiac, paediatrics – the choices are endless. The opportunity to teach and develop other skills is always encouraged within the department.

Cons: None that I can think of, as long as you like a challenge and are not afraid of hard work.

Sub-specialties: Intensive care: for those who like acute medicine. Chronic pain: for those who like outpatients, with a hint of psychology and practical procedures. Trauma: for those who like to pretend they are in ER. Cardiac, neuro, upper and lower GIT surgery and vascular anaesthesia: for those who like sick patients needing invasive monitoring and excellent pain relief. Day case surgery: for those who like fit patients. Orthopaedics and urology: for those who like elderly patients. Then there are management, teaching, risk management, audit and legal/ethical issues.

Allied specialties: Prior to entry to anaesthesia it is positive to do one year in medicine, paediatrics/neonates, ITU or A&E (or combinations). Once into training you will rotate through all the sub-specialties and then develop your chosen sub-specialty in the last two years of training. Whenever you are doing a surgical attachment go into the anaesthetic room and follow the patient through the complete episode – anaesthetic room, theatre and recovery. Your insight into patient care will improve. In terms of electives and work experience just enjoy yourself and see life because it is the ability to talk to patients, inform and reassure them that is essential. Work with the elderly – appreciate their problems and fears. If you are set on a career in anaesthetics do not bother with an F2 job – go for a complementary specialty.

Royal college website address: www.rcoa.ac.uk

Specialty profile: Cardiology

Name: Dr M F Shiu

Position: Consultant Cardiologist

Hospital: University Hospitals Coventry and Warwickshire NHS Trust, Coventry

Daily activities: Average working day is nine hours (excluding travelling). A typical consultant's week consists of: two outpatient clinics, three to five cardiac catheter lab sessions, two ward rounds and a half-day for multi-disciplinary team work. Some ward rounds and clinics have teaching incorporated into them. Remaining time is used for administration, which includes answering patient queries, by phone or letter and dictating letters and discharge summaries.

Qualities required: Cardiology has a number of sub-specialties, suiting many temperaments and skills. Those good with their hands will be suited to coronary interventions. Conversely, you can specialise in imaging and therapeutics, or hypertension if you like the traditions of a physician.

Pros: Job satisfaction is high; mixture of one-to-one patient care and the use of new technology for high-tech imaging and treatment; balance between the one-to-one outpatient work and the group interaction at ward rounds; good mixture of calm elective work and frantic emergencies.

Cons: Long days; the feeling that the rest of the NHS system is not really up to date despite efforts at keeping up with the cutting edge of medicine.

Sub-specialties: Interventional (coronary and other cardiac interventions); imaging (often combined with heart failure); cardiac arrhythmias; cardiovascular medicine (often combined with a general medicine accreditation); grown-up congenital heart disease (a small but important area); academic cardiology (overlaps clinical and basic science).

Allied specialties: A solid general training in acute general medicine is essential. Specialties such as nephrology and ITU give excellent experience with the acutely sick often with multi-system involvement. Overseas electives in Asia, North America and some parts of Africa would provide a good insight into the increasingly global nature of the burden of heart disease and give good preparation for subsequent training.

Royal college website address: www.rcplondon.ac.uk; British Cardiovascular Society (www.bcs.com).

Specialty profile: Ear, Nose and Throat (ENT) Surgery

Name: Mr Paul Wilson

Position: Consultant ENT Surgeon

Hospital: University Hospital of North Staffordshire, Stoke-on-Trent

Daily activities: I am not typical of an ENT surgeon! I undertake a mix of clinics and/ or operating sessions with some administration during lunch or prior to the start of the day. Clinics may be adult or children, and specialty or general.

Qualities required: As with most clinical posts, good communication skills, empathy, good organisation and time management, dexterity.

Pros: On-call generally relaxed, phone queries mainly, family friendly, OK private practice (at present).

Cons: Busy during daytimes and waiting list pressures.

Sub-specialties: Otology, head and neck cancer, thyroid/parathyroid, laryngology and voice, base of skull.

Allied specialties: Plastic surgery, neurosurgery. Begin by asking juniors doing ENT what they think; undertake an elective in ENT; peer work experience at Foundation level as day release.

Royal college website address: www.rcseng.ac.uk

Specialty profile: Endocrinology

Name: Dr Andrew Macleod

Position: Consultant Physician with an interest in diabetes and endocrinology

Hospital: Royal Shrewsbury Hospital, Shrewsbury

Daily activities: I work full-time for the NHS (11 sessions) and also do a small amount of private practice. *Monday*: endocrine clinic, with consultant colleague, SpR, SHO and endocrine nurse. Lunchtime: endocrine meeting. Ward round of acute admissions and occasional evening clinical meetings. *Tuesday*: diabetes clinic (general and young persons), with two clinical assistants; monthly neuropathy clinic. Lunchtime: diabetes meetings; teaching, admin, referrals. Occasional evening: Diabetes UK patient meetings. *Wednesday*: monthly community clinic 34 miles away in Wales; well-supported with local GPs, community diabetes specialist nurse, chiropodists; looking at retinal photographs; radioiodine clinic. Lunchtime: 'grand round'; meetings; catch-up time; occasional ante-natal clinic. *Thursday*: ward round with team; diabetes clinic at another hospital. *Friday*: administration, referrals, planning, discussion with GPs, organisational work, meetings. I am a member of the diabetes and endocrine centre; there is always activity going on; chiropody, diabetes advice and education, retinal screening, dietetics, troubleshooting, endocrine tests, etc.

Qualities required: The ability to put oneself in the position of other people; working well within a team; reaching out into the community; planning whole services; reading the future!

Pros: Diabetes: lots of patient contact; knowing most of the patients in the hospital and people in the Tesco superstore (possibly a con)! Good relationships within diabetes team; advantages of developing better service, close contact with the community and GPs. Diabetes is a common problem, so there are lots of people. Endocrinology: good contrast to diabetes. Rare problems (apart from thyroid, etc.), less people! Fascinating: biochemistry in the human. Simple treatments usually do work and the patients usually get better.

Cons: Time pressure (always more to do with no time); pressure on clinics (patient overload, waiting times, etc.). Trying to organise community services can be frustrating; trying to change patients' lifestyles.

Sub-specialties: Specialist endocrine services: mineral metabolism, adrenal disorders, pituitary disease, obesity, growth, endocrine in pregnancy; diabetes: young persons service, diabetes foot problems, diabetes/obstetric service, diabetic eye disease, impotence, renal/diabetes, neuropathy.

Allied specialties: Any general medical specialty; renal medicine; geriatrics; general practice. Attachment to Diabetes Centre offers exposure to clinics, specialist nurses, dieticians and podiatrists. GP diabetes clinics may also be helpful. Try some endocrinology. General medicine attachment linked to diabetes consultant.

Royal college website address: www.rcplondon.ac.uk

Specialty profile: Forensic Psychiatry

Name: Dr Anne Aboaja

Position: Specialist Registrar in Forensic Psychiatry

Hospital: Arnold Lodge, Leicester

Daily activities: Mornings: communication meeting, ward round or clinical ward work; assessment for court reports or referrals; meetings. Lunchtimes: academic meeting with case presentation or journal club. Afternoons: outpatient clinic at local prison; tribunal; dictating a report or clinical ward work; educational supervision with consultant.

Qualities required: Good oral and written communication skills; non-judgemental approach; ability to work in a team; psychodynamically minded; clear thinker and decisive; empathic; reflective.

Pros: Holistic approach to patient care with the required resources; time to take a thorough history and offer a management plan; helping some of the most socially disadvantaged patients in the NHS; trying to understand the relationship between mental illness and crime; going to court; caring for both mental and physical health; the legal aspects (for example, case law, Mental Health Act, criminal justice system); interesting medicine (for example, treatment-resistant schizophrenia, temporal lobe epilepsy, substance misuse).

Cons: Have to produce long reports; relatively slow admission and discharge rate.

Sub-specialties: Adolescent forensic psychiatry; learning disabilities forensic psychiatry; mental illness forensic psychiatry; women's forensic psychiatry; personality disorder forensic psychiatry; forensic psychotherapy.

Allied specialties: Drugs and alcohol; psychotherapy; general adult psychiatry; rehabilitation psychiatry. Insight into general psychiatry can also be gained in any psychiatric specialty plus some voluntary services such as Nightline. Also getting experience of prison medicine or substance misuse services will help you.

Royal college website address: www.rcpsych.ac.uk

Specialty profile: Gastroenterology

Name: Dr Jayne A Eaden

Position: Consultant Gastroenterologist

Hospital: University Hospitals Coventry and Warwickshire NHS Trust, Warwick

Daily activities: In the morning I have outpatient clinics with my registrar and senior house officer, and we see approximately 30 patients, followed by a lunchtime meeting such as an upper gastrointestinal (GI) multidisciplinary team meeting, discussing cancer patients, planning their treatment and investigations. I may have an endoscopy list (gastroscopies, sigmoidoscopies or colonoscopies) in the afternoon, during which I usually teach my registrar. I will touch base with my juniors at some point during the day if I have not done a formal ward round. After this I may have some referrals to see inpatients on various wards in the hospital. Some sort of evening meeting (e.g. managerial) occurs about once a week.

Qualities required: Enthusiasm; good hand–eye co-ordination; willingness to work hard! You should also be a good listener as some patients cannot be 'cured' of their symptoms (e.g. patients with irritable bowel syndrome) and you have to develop a good rapport in order to work through their problems with them.

Pros: Rewarding; feel like you can make a difference to patients and really affect their prognosis; varied; if you are a 'hands on' practical type of person you will really enjoy doing endoscopies.

Cons: Busy job; demanding; not many females in the country become consultants (about 10% of all gastroenterology consultants) as it is not really regarded as a family-friendly specialty.

Sub-specialties: Can develop a sub-specialty interest into almost any condition affecting the GI tract. Examples are hepatology (liver diseases); inflammatory bowel disease (ulcerative colitis and Crohn's disease); pancreatic conditions; small bowel conditions; nutrition; motility problems; upper GI, such as Barrett's oesophagus, etc.

Allied specialties: GI radiology; GI surgery. You could also try to get involved with some GI research as it would set you aside from other applicants for junior posts, if you can get a paper (or even just an abstract) out of it.

Royal college website address: www.rcplondon.ac.uk British Society of Gastroenterologists (www.bsg.org.uk).

Specialty profile: General and Colorectal Surgery

Name: Mr James Francombe

Position: Consultant General and Colorectal Surgeon

Hospital: University Hospitals Coventry and Warwickshire NHS Trust, Warwick

Daily activities: Ward round, operating, outpatients and endoscopy are the mainstay of my practice. No typical day as weekly timetable changes over an eight-week cycle. Varies, from some weeks being very quiet to very busy during on-call week. Out-of-hours largely limited to on-call, good colleagues cover when not on call.

Qualities required: Hard working; determined; easy to get on with, team player; good communication; sense of humour.

Pros: Work satisfaction; lots of time for family as well as work (depending on timetable); good colleagues; good private practice.

Cons: On-call is stressful; changing timetable.

Sub-specialties: Endoscopy; pelvic floor; incontinence; cancer surgery; inflammatory bowel disease; peri-anal problems.

Allied specialty: Medical gastroenterology. For students with an interest in this specialty it would be a good idea to apply for an attachment to a colorectal surgeon with a good reputation for teaching and quality work. Other aspects to think about before applying for the attachment would be to look at their home life to see the potential work–life balance issues.

Royal college website address: England and Wales (www.rcseng.ac.uk), Edinburgh (www.rcsed.ac.uk).

Specialty profile: General Practice

Name: Dr Tony Lawrence

Position: Principal in General Practice (full-time partner) Surgery: Medical Centre, Lindfield, West Sussex

Daily activities: In the surgery by 7:40 am, booked patients from 8:00 am. One patient will be seen every 10 minutes; surgery until 12 noon, plus extras afterwards (27 or 28 patients seen). Take and make phone calls for 30–40 minutes. House calls or visits; because we are semi-rural we have a high visiting load (I did 1000 consultations in people's homes in 2005). Back to surgery by about 2:15–12:30 pm for either minor operation clinic, diabetes clinic, baby clinic or general appointments. Patients booked no later than 6:30 pm, when the front door is supposed to close. Paperwork at surgery (check letters, results, write referrals, insurance reports, audit, etc.) or I take it home. This is only Monday to Friday as the GP contract excludes Saturday and Sunday.

Qualities required: Sense of humour; good communication skills; reasonable clinical aptitude (you often have to diagnose and treat without the ready availability of complex specialist tests). If you wish to be a partner in general practice then a reasonable sense of business acumen is also essential as you will be running a small business (our five-partner practice turns over several million pounds a year and spends £1.6 million on drugs).

Pros: Independence; huge variety of work; patient-centred; continuity of care over years (generations!); flexibility possible (easy acceptance of part-time and flexible working); close to home; great colleagues; no in-house hospital politics.

Cons: Increasing difficulty in accessing secondary care; increased expectation of the role of primary care in dealing with many issues; quite time-demanding during the week.

Sub-specialties: Clear pathways for development of GPs with special interests working either in secondary care or at primary/secondary boundary.

Allied specialties: Psychiatry; geriatrics; paediatrics; A&E; obstetrics and gynae-cology; well, just about anything really. See the world and experience as wide a diversity of life and medicine as possible – as a GP you will be dealing with anything and everything that walks through the door; the wider your base of experience the more fun the job is.

Royal college website address: www.rcgp.org.uk

Specialty profile: Genitourinary Medicine

Name: Dr Mike Walzman

Position: GUM Consultant

Hospital: George Eliot Hospital, Nuneaton

Daily activities: The specialty is primarily outpatient-based. I spend time within the department on a daily basis doing at least one clinic session per day and sometimes an evening clinic too. The clinical spectrum ranges from sexual health check-ups, diagnosis and management of common sexually transmitted conditions and genital dermatological conditions, to the management of HIV-positive patients. On occasions, I am involved in inpatient management; usually of HIV-positive patients. Apart from doing clinics I have sessions for patient administration, teaching and my own continuing professional development.

Qualities required: Good communication; non-judgemental attitude; ability to put people at ease; good sense of humour!

Pros: The strong team spirit; large and important public health element to the job; dealing primarily with young, healthy patients; often able to give instant reassurance or very quick diagnoses and treatment; do not often have patients die; on-call commitments are usually either negligible or not too arduous; scope to develop a number of 'special interests' within the specialty; as it is a relatively small specialty most consultants will know each other.

Cons: The stigma attached to attending a GUM clinic, which can 'rub-off' onto those working within the specialty; however, nowadays there is very little stigmatisation; patients in general feel comfortable about their attendance and I find that GUM health professionals are in fact highly regarded by colleagues; not generally a specialty for those who are hoping for private practice.

Sub-specialties: HIV; sexual dysfunction; genital dermatology/vulval disorders; psychosexual/psychotherapy. (Apart from HIV, the others would normally be for a special interest clinic and not form a major weekly commitment.)

Allied specialty: Infectious diseases; gynaecology; family planning; dermatology; immunology; virology; microbiology. Student should aim to spend more time (one to two full weeks) in GUM with some time in one or more of the other subspecialties.

Royal college website address: www.rcplondon.ac.uk; British Association for Sexual Health and HIV (www.bashh.org).

Specialty profile: Nephrology

Name: Dr Sara Furness

Position: Specialist Registrar Nephrology and General Internal Medicine

Hospital: Manchester Royal Infirmary, Manchester

Daily activities: Variable. 8:30 am: catch up with paperwork and correspondence. 9:00 am to 2:00 pm: vasculitis and dialysis clinics. Ward rounds last all day: we do not just cover 'pure renal' patients, but look in on shared-care patients all over the hospital, with a large input to ICU and critical care areas. I also see a lot of acute referrals (sometimes five or more a day).

Pros: It is quite a specialised field but needs a good level of general medical knowledge; you get to know your patients and keep track of what happens to them; there is a good mix of clinic work, ward patients and procedures.

Cons: It is quite a controlled specialty (best suited to Type A personalities); long hours; heavy workload.

Qualities required: Organisation and logical thinking; a medical all-rounder; a methodical manner; calmness under pressure; patience.

Sub-specialties: Dialysis medicine; chronic kidney disease (including prevention); vasculitis; transplantation.

Allied specialties: General internal medicine; rheumatology (vasculitis). Try to also spend time with the specialist nurses.

Royal college website address: www.rcplondon.ac.uk

Specialty profile: Neurology

Name: Dr Anthony Kenton

Position: Consultant Neurologist

Hospital: University Hospitals Coventry and Warwickshire NHS Trust, Warwick

Daily activities: Per week I do three outpatient clinics; two to three ward rounds; three to four academic or business meetings; teaching students and administration. But there is no such thing as a typical day!

Qualities required: None are essential! But you must be able to cope with not having quick fixes!

Pros: Interesting diseases; long-term management of patients (e.g. epilepsy, Parkinson's disease); few inpatients so lots of time to discuss cases; on-call is non-resident as a registrar; smallish department so some autonomy; good prospects for teaching students or junior doctors, etc.

Cons: Lots of non-organic disease (dizzy spells, tension headache, etc.); not enough junior grades to run a proper on-call service; lots of pressure on clinic waiting times.

Sub-specialties: Stroke neurology (as I do); multiple sclerosis; movement disorders; epilepsy; nerve/muscle disease; headache; neurorehabilitation.

Allied specialties: Neurophysiology; neurosurgery; neurorehabilitation; psychiatry.

Royal college website address: www.rcplondon.ac.uk

Specialty profile: Obstetrics and Gynaecology

Name: Mr Kim Hinshaw

Position: Consultant Obstetrician and Gynaecologist

Hospital: Sunderland Royal Hospital, Tyne and Wear

Daily activities: My normal clinical work is done from 9:00 am till 5:00 pm Monday to Thursday. The week is varied and includes one major operating list, one alternate weekday case list, one gynaecology outpatient clinic, two ante-natal clinics (including one looking after 'high-risk' obstetric cases), one labour ward session and one obstetric ultrasound clinic (including invasive procedures – amniocentesis, etc.). My interests in undergraduate teaching, research and postgraduate education take up the rest of my week. I have a private gynaecology clinic for a couple of hours after work on a Tuesday – this does not eat into family time too much and pays for the 'extras'!

Qualities required: Enthusiasm, good communication skills and effective team-working are essential as we work with many other disciplines and professionals.

Pros: Day-to-day clinical work is varied; large centres see plenty of interesting clinical cases; supportive department; you are encouraged to develop special interest areas; undergraduate and postgraduate teaching opportunities. The trust is very supportive of my interests outside the immediate clinical area (Chair of the Regional Postgraduate Training Committee and national/international lecturing).

Cons: Frustrations with meeting arbitrary targets that clinicians do not always feel are 'patient friendly'; finding time to fit in clinical work, administration, teaching, lecturing, training, research, family, friends and outside interests! Part of the problem is curtailing my own enthusiasm and making sure my work–life balance is right.

Sub-specialties: Presently, core competencies in both obstetrics and gynaecology are required to become a consultant; eventually consultants orientate to one or the other and develop special interests; in larger hospitals there is often a formal split. Obstetrics: 'high-risk' pregnancy; labour ward management; fetomaternal medicine (including obstetric ultrasound) and maternal medicine. Gynaecology: minimally invasive surgery (laparoscopic and hysteroscopic); infertility; pelvic floor or uro-gynaecology; gynaecological oncology (including colposcopy); gynaecological endocrine/menopause; sexual and reproductive health. Academic: research or teaching is a major component of the job. The future: whether the specialty will totally split is not yet clear. Major changes in gynaecological practice in the last 10 years mean fewer hysterectomies are done for menstrual problems. Generalist consultants of the near future will mainly be an obstetrician and 'office' gynaecologist (will offer emergency gynaecology cover, but will only undertake minor and inter-mediate elective surgery).

Allied specialties: Neonatology/paediatrics; primary care; general medicine; anaesthetics (ITU); general surgery. Electives spent in developing countries are often very productive in terms of hands-on experience in acute obstetrics. It is no longer necessary to undertake formal training outside the specialty in order to become a consultant.

Royal college website address: www.rcog.org.uk

Specialty profile: Oncology

Name: Dr Jane Worlding

Position: Consultant Clinical Oncologist

Hospital: University Hospitals Coventry and Warwickshire NHS Trust, Warwick

Daily activities: Clinic work most days: new patient clinic, outpatients, chemo-therapy clinic, radiotherapy planning and review clinic; weekly ward round; administration.

Qualities required: Good communication skills; patience; empathy; being able to work in a team; an interest in CT, MRI and technical aspects of radiotherapy planning.

Pros: Varied from day to day; good continuity of care for individual patients; technically challenging; technology and computer use involved in radiotherapy planning is enjoyable.

Cons: Can be draining as many patients die eventually.

Sub-specialties: For example, urological, colorectal and skin malignancies; carcinoid tumours.

Allied specialties: Either surgical or physician training complement oncology; radiology would also be useful.

Royal college website address: www.rcplondon.ac.uk

Specialty profile: Orthopaedics

Name: Mr Mohamed Arafa

Position: Consultant Orthopaedic Surgeon; Honorary Clinical Senior Lecturer; Associate Postgraduate Dean

Hospital: The Alexandra Hospital, Redditch (clinical work); Birmingham University (undergraduate); West Midlands Deanery, Birmingham (postgraduate)

Daily activities: I am an early bird! I usually start my pre-operative or postoperative ward round at 7:45 am. I see my secretary to sign letters, respond to correspondence and so on, before going to the theatre or outpatients clinic at 9:00 am. I may have a meeting or a lecture at lunchtime. In the afternoon, I am either in theatre, outpatient clinic or at my office at the West Midlands Deanery. Very important aspects of my daily work are bedside teaching on ward rounds, in outpatient clinics and hands-on training in the operating theatre of the junior doctors. I run my private practice in the evening and the weekend. I spend one to two hours every evening browsing the internet for teaching materials, responding to e-mails and preparing lectures, etc.

Qualities required: Manual dexterity; good hand-eye co-ordination; it is important to posses all the qualities outlined in the GMC guidelines about the duties of a doctor.

Pros: Extremely practical with hands-on approach; highly varied specialty; very rewarding (your efforts will be personally acknowledged by your satisfied patients); excellent opportunity to work in a multi-disciplinary team; challenging and expanding specialty; opportunity for research; has the potential for private practice for those interested.

Cons: Very competitive at entry level; busy on-call rota even as a consultant.

Sub-specialties: Trauma surgery; upper (further divided into shoulder, elbow, wrist and hand surgery) and lower (further divided into hip, knee, ankle and feet surgery) limb surgery, surgical procedures include joint replacement, arthroscopic surgery, ligament reconstruction and correction of congenital deformities; oncological surgery; spinal surgery (deals exclusively with traumatic, degenerative, neoplastic and congenital disorders of the spine).

Allied specialties: Plastic surgery; neurosurgery; A&E; thoracic surgery; general surgery; intensive care; demonstrator of anatomy.

Royal college website address: England and Wales (www.rcseng.ac.uk); Edinburgh (www.rcsed.ac.uk); British Orthopaedic Society (www.boa.ac.uk); Welsh Orthopaedic Society (www.wos.ac).

Specialty profile: Paediatrics

Name: Dr Helen Goodyear

Position: Consultant Paediatrician

Hospital: Heart of England NHS Foundation Trust, Birmingham

Daily activities: There is not really a typical day. We do a week at a time as 'on-take consultant of the week' where all sessions are related to acute clinical care; this is enjoyable but exhausting, in particular in the winter season where over 40 admissions per day are common, including very sick children. The day begins with an hour's administration, signing reports and letters, dealing with general correspondence and e-mails. Clinic is at 9:00 am, which (it is hoped) is finished by 1:00 pm, including letters. We have regular lunchtime meetings. In the afternoon I see patients on the ward, referred for my special interest of paediatric dermatology. I also teach students, perform senior house officer assessments, attend various committees or planning groups, child strategy meetings or conferences and deal with the day's post and e-mails. I often need to phone parents; either to return their call, to give them results or arrange meetings with them for more complex cases.

Qualities required: Must like children and not just babies; be a team worker; have patience; have the ability to listen to both parents and children, and adapt what you are saying so that both can understand; flexibility of approach; good manual dexterity.

Pros: Most children come into hospital unwell, but get better quickly and go home; friendly team-working; great variety.

Cons: More paperwork and less clinical work the more senior that you get; on-call commitments are high even as a senior consultant; emotionally tough when a child dies.

Sub-specialties: There are some recognised sub-specialties, but having a special interest is almost essential for most general paediatricians. However, there are a limited number of posts for tertiary specialists so many find employment as general paediatricians with a special interest.

Allied specialties: General practice; accident and emergency; critical care. Doing your elective abroad, in a developing country: seeing a different aspect of child health; undertaking a paediatric project. Voluntary work with children, there is a wide range possible here so that you are sure that you like being with children. Get a general paediatric student selected component just so that you know what it is like on a paediatric ward. They tend to be much noisier than adult wards. Join the acute admitting team for the week and you will get lots of exposure to children, which is different to do when being taught.

Royal college website address: www.rcpch.ac.uk

Specialty profile: Pathology

Name: Dr Paul Matthews

Position: Consultant Histopathologist, Honorary Senior Lecturer

Hospital: University Hospitals Coventry and Warwickshire NHS Trust, Coventry

Daily activities: Working a rota system with eight other histopathologists, I am responsible for the preparation of complex surgical resection specimens, reporting on histological specimens large and small, reporting on cytological specimens, carrying out autopsies and contributing to multi-disciplinary meetings. I also run modules in Phase 1 and 2 of the Warwick University Medical School graduate entry course. Any one day may involve several or all of these duties, not forgetting some audit and research. Other days might include interviewing prospective medical students or giving evidence at Coroner's Court. I work as part of a team within the department of pathology (e.g. technicians, laboratory staff, secretaries) and as part of clinical teams managing patient care.

Qualities required: A degree of obsessional behaviour; ability to communicate well both verbally and in written form; ability to know your skills and limitations (I often ask a colleague for an opinion); ability to assimilate information from many sources; ability to do three jobs at once (on a quiet day).

Pros: Time to think (unless it's during a frozen section); flexibility to do routine work around other commitments (like answering this questionnaire!); getting close to the elusive, absolute right answer to the question 'What is going wrong with this patient?'(sometimes not possible); working closely with clinicians who listen very closely to what you have to say; a pathologist's opinion may decide whether someone has a radical procedure or toxic chemotherapy; ability to combine routine work with medical school commitments; rarely called in at night.

Cons: Loss of direct patient contact; public perceptions that you only do autopsy work; hardly a glamour specialty; getting very much busier.

Sub-specialties: Almost all pathologists specialise now and have responsibility for one or more sub-specialties. For example, I have an interest in lymphomas and head and neck pathology. Forensics appeals to some while others forsake autopsy work altogether. Some generalisation still happens though. For example, today I have made diagnoses on biopsies from lymph node, tongue, pleura, colon and salivary gland. Variety remains the spice of life.

Allied specialty: Job-wise nothing is a substitute for an F2 post in histopathology. Any clinical experience is a bonus for pathology and any clinical job would benefit from a time in pathology. Go to the mortuary for teaching on clinical aspects of pathology. Follow your patient's biopsy. Seek an elective in pathology, not necessarily in the UK. Turn up for multi-disciplinary meetings and see how pathologists contribute to patient management. Badger a pathologist to run a Special Study Module!

Royal college website address: www.rcpath.org

Specialty profile: Public Health

Name: Dr Stephen Bridgman

Position: DPH/Senior Lecturer

Hospital: Newcastle-under-Lyme Primary Care Trust

Daily activities: Answering e-mails, writing reports, assessing evidence, management (achieving objectives through meetings), trying to progress research projects, representing health service in the media. Loads of out of hours reading required as field of work is so broad. On-call work not very onerous, but when it occurs it can involve thousands of people, be high-profile and take a long time to sort out.

Qualities required: Open to all personalities; must like evaluating things; ability to understand numbers; ability to work and influence people; ability to communicate at individual level and to audience.

Pros: Potential for great influence in shaping health services and making a difference to more than those patients in front of you.

Cons: Difficulty of working with others when you are not in control; political influence.

Sub-specialties: Consultant in communicable disease control; environmental health issues; academic; acute services; primary care.

Allied specialties: A wide range of clinical experience is very helpful, undertake projects in public health topics or shadow public health consultants.

Royal college website address: www.rcplondon.ac.uk

Specialty profile: Radiology

Name: Dr Katharine Foster

Position: Paediatric Radiologist

Hospital: Birmingham Children's Hospital

Daily activities: I typically work from 9:00 am till 5:00 pm, but sometimes I have to arrive earlier for meetings and leave a bit later on other days. We have lists booked each day, so to some extent I know what my day is going to involve, but there are always inpatients and emergencies to be squeezed in. I do CT and plain films on Monday morning, fluoroscopy on Tuesday afternoon, CT and plain films on Wednesday morning, ultrasound Thursday morning and MRI all day Friday. The remaining time is spent at clinical meetings, teaching and catching up with reporting, and talking to other doctors in the hospital about scans and patients.

Qualities required: Fairly meticulous, organised but flexible, able to communicate with colleagues, families and children, a good memory helps, academic in that we spend quite a lot of time looking unusual conditions up in books.

Pros: I see lots of interesting patients, but never have to tell them or their family bad news.

Cons: In many ways, the radiology department is the centre of the hospital; people come down to see you all day to ask you about scans and patients.

Sub-specialties: Paediatric radiology is quite a specialised field already and at BCH we stay very general within that field, as everything needs to be covered on call. Some people have special interests, for example in musculoskeletal radiology. At Great Ormond Street there are more consultants, and hence more specialisation.

Allied specialty: Paediatrics!

Royal college website address: www.rcr.ac.uk

Specialty profile: Respiratory Medicine

Name: Dr Duncan MacIntyre

Position: Consultant Physician in Respiratory and General Medicine

Hospital: Victoria Infirmary, Glasgow

Daily activities: Ward work/rounds (12 hours/week); outpatients (14 hours/ week); investigation work (4 hours/week); patient administration, for example dictation (6 hours/week); general administration, management, audit (8 hours/week); teaching (postgraduate and undergraduate) and clinical meetings (6 hours/week). Average hours for 50-hour week; however, ~55 hours is common.

Qualities required: Reasonable flexibility; empathy with patients who may have chronic diseases or cancer.

Pros: Variety within specialty and general medicine; large patient contact.

Cons: Huge workload is typical.

Sub-specialties: Asthma; lung cancer; sleep apnoea; cystic fibrosis; ventilation; intensive therapy.

Allied specialty: Intensive therapy.

Royal college website address: www.rcplondon.ac.uk

Specialty profile: Rheumatology

Name: Anonymous

Position: Consultant in Medicine and Rheumatology

Hospital: Victoria Infirmary, south side of Glasgow (catchment area population is 200 000)

Daily activities: Ward round, majority are medical patients with some pure rheumatology patients. Dealing with correspondence: signing clinic letters; taking phone calls; going through e-mails. Do rheumatology clinic (three new and six old patients) and discuss some patients seen by 'junior' colleagues. 'Vet' referral letters, dictate letters and read committee papers and other documents.

Qualities required: Hard(ish) working; sense of humour; enjoy multi-professional team-working (some knowledge of rheumatology!).

Pros: There is a degree of self-management and decent pay.

Cons: It can be surprisingly pressurised as a consultant; patients and relatives sometimes seem to feel they own a bit of your soul.

Sub-specialties: Musculoskeletal ultrasound; specific disease-related work (e.g. connective tissue disease, spondylitic disease); science-based work (for example cytokines, immunology, B or T lymphocytes).

Allied specialties: General medicine; immunology; clinical pharmacology. Spend time at a 'pure' rheumatology centre rather than one where much of the workload is general medicine.

Royal college website address: www.rcplondon.ac.uk; British Society for Rheumatology (BSR): www.rheumatology.org.uk

16

Academic medicine: incorporating research and medical education into your career

Research, academia and medical education are crucial for the training of doctors and medical students as well as the progression of medicine as a whole. This chapter shows you how you can incorporate these three components into your career.

Academic medicine is the inclusion of significant amounts of work in the field of research and/or education associated with a university within a clinical medical career. The amount of time you spend doing each aspect of academia and clinical medicine can vary greatly the further through your career that you get. Structured integrated academic clinical training pathways have been introduced over recent years from Foundation Training through to post Certificate of Completion of Training level. In the more junior training grades, academic doctors usually have contracts with an NHS trust and an honorary contract with a university. As doctors progress through Specialty Training and beyond, they may hold full contracts with the university with which they are affiliated and honorary NHS contracts.

The earliest postgraduate opportunity to have to have formal integrated clinical and academic experience is during the Foundation Programme. During an academic Foundation Programme you will spend roughly 25% of your time undertaking academic training and the remaining time undertaking the usual clinical training. The aim of the academic Foundation Programmes are to give trainees a 'taster' of academic medicine to enable them to see if they enjoy it and if they have the potential to do well in an academic career. Information on academic opportunities during the Foundation Programme in the *Operational Framework for Foundation Training*[1] and in the BMA's publication, *A Career in Academic Medicine*[2] including suggested academic outcomes for these experiences, which include participation in a research or educationalist project and development of the skills needed to write a grant proposal. Academic trainees are also expected to meet the usual clinical Foundation competencies expected of non-academic trainees. The Foundation Programme website (www.foundationprogramme.nhs.uk) contains a dedicated page detailing academic Foundation Programme posts and application to these programmes.

The NIHR Coordinating Centre for Research Capacity Development (NCCRCD) now hosts integrated academic clinical training posts, also referred to as Walport posts, which allow trainees who demonstrate potential for academic success to undertake academic training alongside their specialty/GP training. Currently these National Institute for Health Research (NIHR) academic clinical fellowships (ACF) are awarded for three years (or four years if you are undertaking GP training) and during this time you will spend 25% of your time doing academic work. Entry points are currently at Specialty Trainee Year 1 or Year 3 level. With the likely reforms following the Tooke report, ACF posts may coincide with Higher Specialist Training (*see* Chapter 8). Trainees undertaking these posts will hold academic national training numbers (NTN(A)). The intended outcome of the ACF is for you to have developed academic skills, either in research and/or educational methods, as well as having developed an application for a competitive peer-reviewed research training fellowship or educational training programme which would lead to the award of a higher degree.[2] If during your Specialty Training you do not want to continue with your academic training you can change your NTN(A) for a non-academic NTN. If you already have a PhD you may still obtain an ACF post through which you can obtain funding for further research in your area of interest.[2] Further information on the integrated training schemes and application information can be found on the NCCRCD website (www.nccrcd.nhs.uk).

Once you have undertaken your ACF, if you have developed a successful PhD proposal you can go on to undertake either a full time PhD or a part time PhD with the option of incorporating clinical work into your week as well. Further structured integrated clinical and academic posts are then available should you want to take your academic activities higher. See the NCCRCD website for further information (www.nccrcd.nhs.uk).

The formal academic training schemes are the most streamlined and structured ways of gaining academic experience early on in your clinical career. They enable trainees to dip in and out of academic experience as they wish. For example, you can use an academic Foundation training post as a taster to see if you would like to pursue an academic career further. If so you could apply for an NCCRCD integrated academic training post in the specialty of your choice. If not, you can leave academia to one side, join a normal Specialty Training programme and consider taking academic medicine up again in the future. If you are not successful in being awarded a formal academic training post, or you decide later in your career that you want to enter into academic medicine, there are multiple organisations through which you can obtain funding and support to do this. *The Gold Guide* describes academic options for doctors in Specialty Training posts.[3] Further details of funding and academic opportunities can be found on the following websites: NIHR (www.nihr.ac.uk), Medical Research Council (www.mrc.ac.uk) and the Wellcome Trust (www.wellcome.ac.uk).

Academic medicine allows you to increase your knowledge base and skills in such a way that all aspects of your work are mutually complemented. See Figure 16.1 as an illustration of how clinical medicine, research and education training are mutually beneficial. Academic medicine has become more financially favourable with the introduction of the integrated clinical training posts. Although your pay may be limited by reduced numbers of unsociable hours worked, the basic salary is usually comparable with your non-academic colleagues, but check this out before you apply to an academic post.

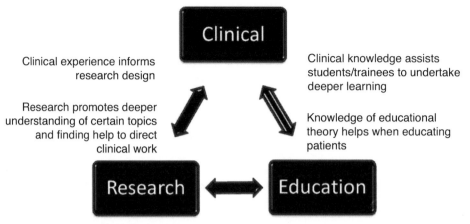

Clinical experience informs research design

Research promotes deeper understanding of certain topics and finding help to direct clinical work

Clinical knowledge assists students/trainees to undertake deeper learning

Knowledge of educational theory helps when educating patients

Knowledge gained through research can enrich skills in education

Educational knowledge and experience can help to disseminate research findings

FIGURE 16.1 How clinical, research and education work mutually benefit each other

If you want to apply to one of the integrated clinical and academic posts you must be aware that often the application processes are opened in advance of the solely clinical training posts application processes. Therefore, you must check the Foundation Programme website or the NCCRCD website as appropriate for up to 6 months before the general application processes open.

Before you apply to an academic training post be clear about the way in which it will be delivered. For example, you will need to think about your preferences and seek out the appropriate programmes with regard to the following.

● Academic focus – research or education? Only very few integrated programmes focus on medical education, most are research posts. If you want to undertake research, you should decide what type of research you are most interested in gaining experience in. For example, the options include lab-based research, qualitative research, educational research or clinical research. Each is wildly different in both the experience you will get and the skills you will gain.

● Delivery of academic component. In some places the academic component is delivered as a solid block of time and in others the academic time is spread across a number of months so that you will be undertaking one to three days of academic training a week.

● Your future intended career. It is essential that you find posts that will help you get to where you want to be. For example, if you know you want to go into medical education, apply to an academic post that incorporates a medical education element, or one that can be further developed in the future to incorporate medical education.

As an academic clinician you may encounter a few drawbacks. You will be undertaking two demanding jobs. Although the academic work usually occurs in a more controlled environment, both clinical and academic work carry their own stressors and you may hit a busy period with both at the same time. On occasions it may feel as if you are doing the equivalent of two jobs. Do not let this put you off. However, you must not think that undertaking an academic training post or career path is an easy option.

As an academic trainee you must be conscious that you will have to complete the same clinical competencies as your peers who are not undertaking any academic work. In certain circumstances (e.g. academic Foundation training), this may result in you having to achieve the same competencies in less time. This is entirely possible; however, you have to plan your learning and be more conscious of getting your assessments done in a timely fashion than your non-academic colleagues.

Sometimes academic and clinical commitments clash. Therefore you will need to have built a good, trusting and respectful relationship with your colleagues and supervisors to be able to negotiate required time away from your usual scheduled activities. This can usually be done without a problem, providing you are making up the time away elsewhere and clinical service provision is not affected.

It is well worth speaking with people who have previously undertaken the post(s) you are considering applying for as they will be able to inform you of the benefits and pitfalls of the post you are interested in. In addition, they will help you to understand the nature of academic medicine as it is a concept many students and junior doctors struggle to comprehend and thus may miss out on chances to undertake a different strand of medicine they may otherwise enjoy and excel at.

If you are awarded an academic training post, make sure you make early contact with the university with which you are affiliated. You will need to arrange access to computer and library facilities as soon as possible to prevent time wasted. If you have any problems arranging this you should speak as soon as you can with your academic supervisor.

The rest of this chapter will explain further about the types of academic work and the ways in which you can experience and incorporate academic components into your career.

RESEARCH IN YOUR CAREER

Research is performed in order to improve medical practice. You can take part in research at any point in your career. Examples of research opportunities include intercalated degrees and case studies. Research is an important part of any modern health system that values evidence-based medicine.[4]

There are several good reasons for you to do research, including:[4]

- improving your understanding of research techniques that will better enable you to critically interpret and understand published work
- starting a career-long involvement in research, either as a leader or as a member of a team
- as part of your training; for example, to become an academic consultant.

If you are involved in research to complement what you foresee as a purely clinically role, it is sensible to focus on the specialty in which you wish to work.[4] If you intend to have a more academic career then the quality of the research is more important than the topic.[4]

Published research will enhance your CV, and thus your future job applications. Simply performing research does not automatically mean it will be published.[5] To increase the chances of getting your work published it should address a subject of interest to the editors (and readers) of the journals you decide to send it to and it must be of good quality.[5] Good research takes time, so you will require good time-management skills.[5]

The department in which you complete your research usually funds your studies. The department, in turn, receives financial support from research funding bodies or industry.[4] You can obtain funding from personal research training fellowships.[4] These are more desirable and are awarded in open competition after peer review of a grant application that may be offered by the Medical Research Council (MRC), research charities or industry,[4] as described above.

MEDICAL EDUCATION IN YOUR CAREER

As with other academic medicine, there is no specific career route into medical education. To assist your career path in becoming a medical educator you can undertake various courses to improve your teaching skills or knowledge of medical education; for example, certificates, diplomas or masters in medical education. You may even undertake research in relation to medical education.

You can combine a career in medical education with another in medical academia; however, the two careers are not synonymous. There are potentially four reasons why you may want to be involved in medical education.

1 To improve your skills in teaching juniors and students, or to become a student tutor or mentor.
2 To work in a local postgraduate deanery as a GP tutor, course organiser or clinical tutor.
3 To become a senior managerial figure in medical education; for example, a senior lecturer in a medical school or postgraduate dean.
4 To improve the education of medics via research; for example, developing new learning methods like problem-based learning.

The Association for the Study of Medical Education (ASME) website (www.asme. org.uk) is a good place to gain further information. In addition, a few ACF posts are designed to train you in medical education rather than research so if you have a real interest in medical education, seek these scarce posts out.

Specialty profile: Academic Medicine

Name: Professor Ruth Chambers

Position: Director of Postgraduate General Practice Education at West Midlands Deanery, Professor of Primary Care at Staffordshire University, GP.

Where have you carried out your research? 1988: part-time research fellow at Keele University, progressing to be part-time senior lecturer. 1995: completed my MD (Doctorate) thesis, which I gained from the University of Nottingham. 1997: Professor of Primary Care at Staffordshire University. I have teams of staff to work on research and development projects with me. I work with academics from other institutions across the UK and overseas and with colleagues from different specialties at my own university. Throughout I have remained as a GP, working full-time until 1997, and since then for one or two sessions per week.

Daily activities: Attracting research funding; agreeing the research and development protocol; applying for ethics and research governance approval; appointing the team and generally overseeing that we are fulfilling the research protocol; writing up research for a peer-reviewed journal.

Qualities required: Self-belief in your ability is vital; a wide base of knowledge and skills; the ability to teach; good communication skills.

Opportunities: You can make academic medicine your main career or a fringe activity, work with the royal college of your specialty, travel the world, use your research or teaching materials to write books. I have done all of these and am now on my 58th book.

Advice to interested students: Gain experience by helping the research department in your teaching hospital gather data as part of an ongoing research study.

REFERENCES

1 Department of Health. *Operational Framework for Foundation Training.* UK Foundation Programme Office; 2007. Available at: www.foundationprogramme.nhs.uk/pages/home/key-documents (accessed 15 January 2009).
2 British Medical Association Academic Staff Committee. *A Career in Academic Medicine.* London: British Medical Association; 2006.
3 Department of Health. *A Reference Guide for Postgraduate Specialty Training in the UK.* 2nd ed. London: Department of Health; 2008. Available at: www.mmc.nhs.uk/default.aspx?page=457 (accessed 8 February 2009).
4 Weissberg P. Research in clinical training. *BMJ Career Focus.* 2002; **325**: 97.
5 Albert T. Publish and prosper. *BMJ Career Focus.* 1996; **313**: 2.

FURTHER READING

Academic Medicine Group. *Guidelines for Clinicians Entering Research.* London: Royal College of Physicians; 1997.
British Medical Association. Academic medicine in the NHS: driving innovation and improving healthcare. 2008. Available at: www.bma.org.uk/careers/careers_academic_medicine/AcademicmedicineNHS.jsp (accessed 8 February 2009).
British Medical Association. *Medical Academic Career Intentions: results of the BMA cohort study of 1995 medical graduates.* London: British Medical Association; 2004.
British Medical Association. *Role Models in Academic Medicine.* London: British Medical Association; 2005. Available at: www.bma.org.uk/employmentandcontracts/recruitment/Rolemodels.jsp

British Medical Association. *Women in Academic Medicine: challenges and issues*. 2004. Available at: www.bma.org.uk/employmentandcontracts/equality_diversity/gender/womenacademic.jsp

British Medical Association Medical Education Sub-committee of the Board of Science. *Medical Specialties: the way forward*. London: British Medical Association; 2007.

Research Capacity Development Programme (www.nccrcd.nhs.uk)

Royal College of Physicians. *Clinical Academic Medicine: the way forward*. London: Royal College of Physicians; 2004. (Aimed at those engaged in medical education and research, this report contains clinical academic pathways with explanations of specific details for each discipline.)

GPs with a special interest

The potential roles of GPs are changing; one of these changes is to develop GPs with a 'special interest' (GPwSI). This chapter details how you may become a GP with a special interest, the benefits of this and what it involves.

The Department of Health has defined a GPwSI as:

> '[A GP who supplements] their core generalist role by delivering an additional high quality service to meet the needs of patients. Working principally in the community they deliver a clinical service beyond the scope of their core professional role or may undertake advanced interventions not normally undertaken by their peers. They will have demonstrated appropriate skills and competencies to deliver those services without direct supervision.'[1]

GPwSIs have developed an additional expertise that expands their clinical practice in a specific field.[2] The rationale and duties of a GPwSI are not the same as GPs who work as hospital practitioners or clinical assistants in hospital or other settings. Nor are they expected to be equivalent to consultants in the corresponding specialty in respect of their caseload. Indeed, GPwSIs work with the support and oversight of hospital consultants in order to provide a wider range of outpatient or community based services. These may include minor surgery and diagnostic procedures.

There is a trend to shift the care of patients from hospital to primary care and establishing GPwSIs supports this.[3] Increasingly, it is recognised that other healthcare workers can have more specialist roles, thus guidance is being implemented that encompasses dentists, pharmacists, nurses and other allied health professionals. Therefore the term Practitioners with Special Interests (PwSI) is now more commonly used.[4] Through having PwSI in the locality, patients are able to access services more easily, both more quickly and more conveniently, with more choice in their management.

The appointment of a PwSI will only occur when a review of the local health and service provision is performed, priorities are identified and the need for specialist services is agreed.[5] Therefore, you cannot expect to obtain a GPwSI post just because you are adequately qualified. The national framework for GPwSIs was initially launched in 2002; this was revised in 2007 and is laid out in Part 3 of the document, *Implementing Care Closer to Home: convenient quality of care for patients.*[1] This Department of Health publication sets out the common set of principles that all PwSIs should have:[4]

- the ability to drawn on generalist skills and expertise in order to play role of gatekeeper to more specialist services in a particularly effective way
- the ability to act without direct supervision
- the level of skill or competence required to deliver the service that exceeds the core competencies of the individuals normal professional role
- an appropriate qualification – although qualification alone does not demonstrate suitability for the role.

GPwSI have been put into posts, and frameworks exist in the following mainstream specialty areas:
- cardiology
- care for older people
- child protection
- dermatology
- diabetes
- drug misuse
- ear, nose and throat (ENT)
- endoscopy
- epilepsy
- headache
- learning disability
- mental health
- pain management
- palliative care
- respiratory disease
- sexual health (as part of women's and child health)
- urgent and emergency care.

Specialty specific guidance is available on the Primary Care Contracting website (www.pcc.nhs.uk/245.php). Other specialties in which GPs have developed special interests when a need has been identified, include:
- care of those who find access to traditional health services difficult (e.g. the homeless, asylum seekers, travellers)
- musculoskeletal medicine
- ophthalmology
- orthopaedics
- other procedures suitable for a community setting (e.g. vasectomies).

As a GPwSI, your priority is to continue as a generalist, but spend about two sessions a week practising your specialty. The benefits to you, as a GPwSI, include lower 'did not attend' (DNA) rates at clinics and structured professional development and education.[3,6] You would be required to set aside a prescribed number of hours for continuing professional development each year to remain up-to-date in your specialty field. You should also keep and maintain a portfolio to demonstrate the competencies you have acquired and sustained. You can expect to be assessed and revalidated on a regular basis. Depending on the PCT appointing you, various accreditation schemes are available including diplomas and local accreditation or certification schemes. Accreditation and appointment is outlined in Part 3 of *Implementing Care Closer to Home: Convenient Quality of Care for Patients.*[1]

REFERENCES

1 Department of Health. *Implementing Care Closer to Home: convenient quality of care for patients. Part 3: The accreditation of GPs and pharmacists with special interests.* London: Department of Health publications; 2007. Available at: www.dh.gov.uk/en/Publicationsandstatistics/Publications/PublicationsPolicyAndGuidance/DH_074428 (accessed 15 January 2009).

2 Department of Health. *Practitioners with Special Interests: bringing services close to patients.* London: Department of Health Publications; 2003.

3 Royal College of General Practitioners. *General Practitioners with Special Interests.* 2004. Available at: www.rcgp.org.uk (accessed 15 January 2009).

4 Department of Health. *Implementing Care Closer to Home: convenient quality of care for patients. Part 1: introduction and overview.* London: Department of Health publications; 2007. Available at: www.dh.gov.uk/en/Publicationsandstatistics/Publications/PublicationsPolicyAndGuidance/DH_074428 (accessed 15 January 2009).

5 Department of Health. *Implementing a Scheme for General Practitioners with Special Interests.* 2002. Available at: www.dh.gov.uk/PublicationsAndStatistics/Publications/PublicationsPolicyAndGuidance/DH_4009799 (accessed 8 February 2009).

6 Department of Health. *New Roles for Nurses and GPs to Expand Primary Care and Drive Down Waiting Lists.* 2003. Available at: www.dh.gov.uk/PublicationsAndStatistics/PressReleases/DH_4024519 (accessed 8 February 2009).

FURTHER READING

Association of Practitioners with Special Interests (http://apwsi.co.uk/)

Baker M and Chambers R. *A Guide to General Practice Careers.* London: Royal College of General Practitioners; 2000.

Primary Care Contracting website. (section on Practitioners with Special Interests www.pcc.nhs.uk/173.php)

18

Working abroad

Up to 60% of doctors who are one year post-graduation plan to practise medicine outside the UK. For the majority of cases this is on a temporary basis, to increase life experience, get the opportunity to travel and to broaden medical experience.[1] However, arranging to work abroad is a complex process. There are many aspects to take into consideration: visas, indemnity, exams, registration, immigration issues, the crime situation – let alone a job to go to and accommodation. This chapter gives you a brief overview of the aspects you should be aware of, or investigate further, before you embark on medical student, or postgraduate work or training abroad.

If you have never thought about working abroad before, there are several aspects you should consider. Think why you would want to do so and what you would want to get out of the experience. People often decide to work abroad for personal reasons: for a change of pace, maybe to escape from any pressures of home or work, to take unique opportunities, to have greater personal responsibility or just to have some fun. You may want to develop your clinical skills, experience medicine in another culture, go for the teaching, achieve something specific or to stand out from other doctors when it comes to developing your CV. Increasingly, junior doctors are spending a year abroad before embarking on their Specialty Training.

Think *where* you might want to work; in a developed or less-developed country. If you want to work in third-world countries, especially for voluntary organisations, they prefer doctors with a reasonable amount of experience rather than relatively junior trainees. There, you are given a lot more responsibility, although conditions may be poor and equipment is often lacking. Do you want to experience Western medicine or maybe traditional Tibetan, Chinese or Outback medicine? If you need to be paid you should go to a developed country.

Think *when* you would like to work abroad. It is common to complete the Foundation Programme before working abroad. The more junior you are, the less experience you have, but you are also less established in that you are less likely to have a mortgage, children and significant other to keep you in the UK. If you are working overseas later in your career, think about the skills that would be most valuable. For instance, surgical and anaesthetic skills are often extremely useful in third-world countries or in emergency situations such as disaster relief.

Following is information on working abroad, with specific information where appropriate. This information is a rough guide to what you should think about if planning to work or train abroad. Before you travel you must make sure you research the information provided to make sure it is up to date.

HOW POPULAR IS YOUR DESIRED DESTINATION?

Certain destinations are very popular, especially for medical student electives. Therefore, aside from all the arrangements that you have to make in advance, it is a really good idea to start planning your time abroad as early as possible. It is recommended that if you want to study in a popular destination, such as the USA, you should apply at least one year in advance.

WHAT DOCUMENTATION AND PERMISSIONS ARE REQUIRED BEFORE YOU CAN WORK AT YOUR DESIRED DESTINATION?

Following the Council Directive 75/362/EEC, passed in 1975, and subsequent European Union Council Directives (e.g. 93/16/EEC available to read from http://ec. europa.eu/internal_market/qualifications/specific-sectors_doctors_en.htm) there has been mutual recognition of medical qualifications with the result that doctors can move freely between Austria, Belgium, Denmark, Finland, France, Germany, Greece, Iceland, Ireland, Liechtenstein, Luxembourg, The Netherlands, Norway, Portugal, Spain, Sweden and the UK. You are entitled to full registration in any European Union (EU) country if you are a citizen of a member state and have completed primary training in a member state, obtaining a recognised qualification. However, as part of the registration process, most authorities or councils require:

- a medical degree certificate
- a Certificate of Completion of Training (CCT) or vocational training (VT) certificate
- passport
- certificate of good standing
- a CV
- a certificate of good health or medical fitness to practise
- evidence of ability to speak the native language.

Each of the above may require translation into the country's native language.

For some countries out of the EU, you may be required sit additional exams, for example, the United States Medical Licensing Examination (www.usmle.org) and the Australian Medical Council exams (if you haven't completed specialist training; www.amcexams.com/examdetails.htm). Make sure you research the prospect of this early to give yourself enough time to apply, study and pass the exam in time for your planned departure.

Often if you are travelling as a student to another country for a short placement or elective, especially within the European Economic Area (EEA), visas and registration are not required. However, you must investigate this while you plan your placement. If a visa is required, either as a student or for working doctors, you must allow a long time for the visa application to be processed. Visas are usually awarded on a points basis: if you are wishing to apply to a country which is actively seeking medically trained professionals you will be awarded more points and would thus be more likely to be successful in your visa application. One example of such a country has been

Australia; however, as workforce patterns change this may do also.

Information on entry requirements for travel to each country around the world can be obtained from the Foreign and Commonwealth Office (FCO) website (www. fco.gov.uk)

As with any trip abroad, don't forget to make sure you hold a 10-year passport and that there is adequate time left on this. Some countries require you to have at least 6 months left on your passport. Another important set of documents to arrange is travel insurance. Make sure you have adequate cover and be careful to read the small print. If you are planning to undertake any dangerous activities, such as snowboarding, you need to make sure this is also covered.

ARE THERE ANY PERSONAL SAFETY AND HEALTH ISSUES YOU MUST CONSIDER?

You may have to address some health issues before you go to work in certain countries. For some destinations a certificate of good health may be all that is required, for others you may require a chest x-ray (e.g. Australia), or proof of hepatitis B immunity (e.g. USA).

Infectious diseases (e.g. TB and malaria), are a significant medical problem in certain areas, such as Africa. Therefore, you must consult your practice nurse or GP well in advance to arrange the appropriate immunisations. Also, in some areas of Africa (e.g. Zimbabwe), HIV seropositivity is as high as 60% so you must be careful when carrying out invasive procedures. You should also speak with a medical professional, ideally an infectious diseases consultant, before you go about taking post-exposure prophylaxis in the event that you think you have been exposed to HIV.

If you are travelling within EEAs you may be entitled to free or discounted medical care. To be able to qualify you will need to carry a free European Health Insurance Card (EHIC). For details on where to obtain one, visit www.dh.gov.uk/travellers.

In terms of personal safety, you must consider the prevalence of crime and political instability in the area you want to work in. As a first point of reference you should visit the FCO website (www.fco.gov.uk) in order to gain information about country-specific travel, including those countries or areas of countries you are advised against travelling to. The FCO website also contains more detailed information on staying safe and healthy while abroad, being a responsible tourist and what to do if things go wrong.

WHAT CULTURAL ISSUES AND CUSTOMS MUST YOU CONSIDER?

Cultural expectations and norms are different in every country across the world. The issues may be different depending on whether you are male or female and even your sexual preferences. If you are not aware of the cultural issues of the country you are working in and do not try to fit in with cultural norms you may not only alienate yourself, but also cause offence and potentially attract the attention of local authorities and/or police. For example, showing too much flesh or keeping your shoes on in the wrong circumstances can be a terrible misdemeanour. If you are travelling to an area predominantly populated by individuals following a certain religion, there will be an expectation that you conform to their customs to some extent. For example, in mainly Muslim countries you should respect the custom of fasting between sunrise and sunset during Ramadan. Acceptance of homosexual relationships has improved in many places compared with the past, but public displays of affection between same-sex couples can lead to negative attention from police and local authorities (e.g. in Cuba), and potentially homophobic related crimes (e.g. in New Zealand). More mundane offences, such as crossing a road or tram track within 50 m of a designated crossing point, may land you with a fine if you are travelling to the Czech Republic, and changing money on the streets rather than in an exchange shop, bank or hotel is illegal in Romania.

A wealth of useful information, including all of the above is found on the FCO website.

HOW WILL YOU PROTECT YOURSELF PROFESSIONALLY?

If you are going to be working abroad you must obtain professional indemnity to protect yourself. The main medical defence organisations, such as the Medical Protection Society and the Medical Defence Union, do provide cover in certain situations. Make sure you contact your indemnity organisation well in advance to obtain quotes and arrange cover.

WHAT ARE THE TRAINING ISSUES FOR JUNIOR DOCTORS?

The BMA advises that you do not spend time working abroad until you have completed the generic training of the Foundation Programme.[2] If you do not want to heed to this advice you must make sure with the GMC that the training you will get abroad will lead to full UK registration and you need to find out if the PMETB will recognise your training.[2]

Many doctors, at the time of print, choose to travel abroad between Foundation and Specialty Training. In effect they are taking a year out of the training pathway and postpone their application to Specialty Training for when they get back. If this is what you want to do, don't forget that you will have to budget and factor in travel and time off for travel to interviews in the UK should your Specialty Training applications be successful while you are away.

The BMA guidance on working abroad provides the options on gaining time out of Specialty Training to work abroad.[2]

HOW CAN WORKING ABROAD BE MADE EASIER?

As more and more junior doctors travel abroad for at least a year to experience the health service elsewhere, organisations and agencies are arising to make the arrangements for travel a lot easier. For example, if you are planning to work in the developed world, MedRecruit (www.medrecruit.com) and International Medical Recruitment (IMR; www.imrmedical.com) are both sources of help for junior doctors wishing to travel to New Zealand and/or Australia, and Alberta, Canada (www.albertacanada.com/immigration/campaigns/doctors.html) is a site that assists doctors wishing to work in Alberta, Canada. It is well worth identifying relevant agencies and/or organisations for both paid and/or voluntary work abroad as they will have knowledge and experience from people who have gone before you. Just beware that negative testimonials are unlikely to be found on these organisations' websites, so make sure you carefully consider the pros and cons independently.

If you would like to work in the developing world, many doctors join in with established aid agencies rather than arranging jobs themselves.[2] Be sure to pick the agencies that suit your personal requirements and commitments.[2] Examples of such agencies include, Médecins Sans Frontières (www.msf.org.uk) and Voluntary Service Overseas (www.vso.org.uk).

The International Department of the BMA has produced two guides for doctors planning to move to and work abroad[2] and, specifically, in the EEA and Switzerland.[3] The former guide provides information on planning a temporary career move abroad, returning to the NHS and information on working the developed and developing world. The latter guide is essential reading for any doctor planning a move within the EEA as it covers, among other important topics, legislation around working in the EEA, required language competences, how to find a permanent or temporary post and a section devoted to finding work in each EEA country. The guide also contains many useful web links to follow for each country. Contact the International Department of the BMA directly if you need information on registration and practice in other countries. Contact details of the International Department as well as free access to the guides are available through the BMA website (www.bma.org.uk).

A FINAL WORD OF ADVICE

In general, plan early. Consider the language, climate, nature and extent of infectious diseases, and state of the healthcare system where you are going – and think of your personal safety. Try to arrange to have a job to come back to before you go. This may involve making an application and succeeding in an interview before you leave.

REFERENCES

1 British Medical Association. *The Cohort Study of 2006 Medical Graduates.* 2nd report. British Medical Association: London; 2008.
2 British Medical Association. *Guide to Working Abroad.* London: British Medical Association; 2007.
3 British Medical Association. *Opportunities for Doctors within the European Economic Area.* London: British Medical Association; 2006.

FURTHER READING

British Medical Association Medical Education Sub-Committee of the Board of Science. *Medical Specialties: the way forward.* London: British Medical Association; 2007.
Wilson M. *The Medic's Guide to Work and Electives around the World.* London: Arnold Publishers; 2000.

Diverse medical careers

19

You may not have considered all the weird and wonderful career options available to you as a doctor. This chapter will give you a taste of some of the careers you may not have thought of yet.

WORKING IN THE DEFENCE SERVICES

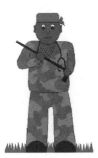

The defence services consist of the Army,[1] Royal Air Force[2] and Royal Navy.[3] Entry can occur from medical student level onwards. The first three years after graduation involves both medical and defence service training. Although differences occur in careers in each military service, this section will give a general idea of what you may expect. It is up to you to get more specific information.

Many disciplines are available in the defence services; from A&E to otorhinolaryngology and anaesthetics to ophthalmology. As in civilian medicine, selection depends upon academic ability and the availability of jobs.

The advantages of working in the defence services are well advertised. Generous bursaries, cadetships and payment of tuition fees are available to medical students. After graduation, the salary compares favourably with that of civilian doctors. Aside from the monetary gains, you can experience the world, gain leadership and management skills, and learn how to cope with the unpredictable.

Disadvantages of a career in the defence services are not so well known, but it is important to consider them carefully. The job is unpredictable: you may be contacted with little or no prior warning to be sent anywhere in the world on service, exercises or on peace keeping and humanitarian operations. You are unlikely to be sent to glamorous places; you can expect to spend time in devastated and dangerous areas. Thus, progress in postgraduate training can be delayed.

Although you are likely to be rich compared with many of your medical school peers, wealth does not come without ties. You will be obligated to serve for at least six years after graduation. Unfortunately, you can never tell how your life may change during medical school, as it is a time when you may go through great personal development. Money may not compensate you for this obligation if your circumstances change.

A survey carried out by the BMA of over 200 defence service doctors, covering the three military services, showed that nearly half worked over 50 hours per week.

141

In addition, more than 50% were not able to take their full annual leave entitlement and nearly 10% had spent more than 100 days in deployment on active service over the previous year.[4]

PRISON DOCTOR

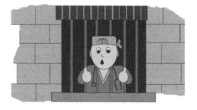

There are a number of openings for GPs to work within the prison medical service, which has only recently become part of the NHS.[5] The Royal Colleges of General Practitioners (RCGP), Physicians (RCP) and Psychiatrists (RCPsych) have designed a diploma in prison medicine. Prison healthcare officers, nurses and pharmacists will support your work. In addition, visiting specialists, such as psychiatrists, dentists and optometrists, may hold clinics in prisons.[6]

As patients, the majority of inmates are needy. Many come from deprived backgrounds and they are often homeless. Therefore, other than routine medical screening of new inmates and GP work, a prison doctor's caseload often involves the management of problems common to many prisoners: mental health problems, substance misuse and communicable diseases. In addition, as their advocate, you should ensure that the conditions of detention are not having a deleterious effect on their health – either mental or physical. Drawbacks of this career include possible demands by prison staff and authorities that could conflict with your ethical obligations. It is important that you are aware of this so you can manage such situations appropriately.

SHIP'S DOCTOR

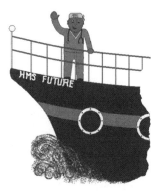

Does sailing the seas while trying to save lives (!) appeal to you? Being a ship's doctor,[7] you will have the opportunity to experience more of the world and its people. Being able to communicate well and being sociable are essential.

If you choose to work on a cruise liner you can expect very well-equipped facilities. Many such vessels have onboard x-ray facilities, an ITU, mini-laboratory for testing blood, pharmacy, a treatment room that doubles up as an operating theatre and several wards for inpatients.

Contracts may be four to eight months in length. Depending on the size of the ship, and the number of doctors, you will be expected to run one or two clinics a day. All patients are seen on a private basis; therefore some will be more demanding and will require a more tolerant attitude. If uniforms do not 'float your boat' you need to think of another career. Expect to wear an officer's uniform whenever you are near passenger areas.

The most essential training experience you would need is in general practice.

You should also have had rotations in A&E and had experience on ITU. For some jobs you are required to have at least three years' experience in emergency medicine. Other useful areas to experience during your training would be general medicine, care of the elderly and psychiatry. In addition, you must also have gained an advanced cardiac life support certificate. If you are planning on being a doctor on a ship with American passengers you will also be required to complete the advanced trauma life support course.

MEDIA DOCTOR

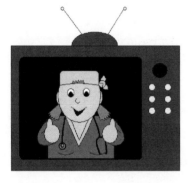

Being a media doctor may be the career for you if you enjoy explaining things clearly. You can be a media doctor in various ways: writing (including technical work), radio, television and the Internet. It can be fun and a chance to communicate with many people.

However, becoming a media doctor is not easy, and being successful is even harder. Initially, many write for papers and magazines. You can move on from writing comments, to features, articles, health columns or even books.

Getting on radio and television is even more difficult. There are few openings and, as anything can be thrown at you, you require training in both medical and media skills. You also need to be engaging, something which may not come naturally to you.[8]

As a media doctor, you cannot guarantee when each job will arise and you can expect to get limited time for preparation. However, it is possible to practise part-time medicine whilst being in the media, to provide some stability.

Not everyone will agree with what you do. As a media doctor, not only are you leaving yourself open for misrepresentation, you are exposing yourself to potential hostility from patients, the public and even your colleagues.[9]

MEDICINE AND THE LAW

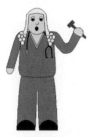

Only a few careers accommodate both medicine and law:[10] a coroner and regulatory work within the pharmaceutical industry. However, if you are already a doctor, but would like to work in a legal-related field there are a number of options, including forensic pathology, forensic psychiatry, police surgeon, prison doctor, medical adviser for a medical defence organisation or court or other legal professions and academics in forensic medicine, forensic sciences or medical law and ethics. Generally, once you have completed two years as a specialist registrar, you can concentrate on one of the specialties mentioned above. It is possible to obtain a diploma in forensic medicine or law. However, as a doctor you are unlikely to get financial support to study for a legal qualification.

Skills required include the ability to explain technical information in a concise manner understandable to lay people. You should also have the confidence to handle widely publicised cases and to withstand harsh cross-examination in court.

PREMIER LEAGUE DOCTOR

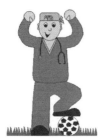

You want football to be your life and being a doctor will be your life, so why not combine the two? It is not difficult to see the drawbacks of wanting to be a premier league doctor,[11,12] not least the number of premier league teams there are across the country. Therefore, setting your sights on sports medicine in local teams may be best initially. The principle is the same and, who knows, you might get lucky.

GP training is the usual starting block, followed by a diploma in sports medicine. Rotations during training should include general medicine and A&E. Other useful placements would be rheumatology and orthopaedics. Once trained, GPs are expected to spend at least half their time dedicated to sports and exercise medicine to be deemed competent. As a premier league doctor you would be spending 100% of your time working in sports medicine.

Good experience can be gained by working and volunteering with local teams; however, you must have appropriate training otherwise you will not be protected against litigation.

Life as a premier league doctor is not all glamorous. You would be on call around the clock and have to travel everywhere that the team goes. If musculoskeletal examination is not your forte you would have to work hard to change this or think again. Currently, sports medicine is not recognised by the royal colleges as a specialty in its own right. However, several UK universities offer diplomas in sports medicines.

REFERENCES

1 Royal Army Medical Corps. *What Does Army Medicine Involve?* Available at: http://armyjobs. haymarketnetwork.com/images/pdf/hi_AOF0055.pdf (accessed 15 January 2009).
2 Royal Air Force Careers. *Medical Officers.* Available at: www.rafcareers.com/jobs (accessed 8 February 2009).
3 Royal Navy. *Medical Officer.* Available at: www.royalnavy.mod.uk/server/show/nav.6067 (accessed 8 February 2009).
4 British Medical Association. *Armed Forces Doctors' Pay Rise Fails to Address Recruitment and Retention Crisis.* 26 May 2005. Available at: www.bma.org.uk (accessed 15 January 2009).
5 Aquino P and Jones P. *Career Options in General Practice.* Oxford: Radcliffe Publishing; 2004.
6 Longfield M. Opportunities for doctors in the prison service. *BMJ Career Focus.* 1999; **318**: 2.
7 Shafi S. Working as a ship's doctor. *BMJ Career Focus.* 1998; **316**: 2.
8 Easton G. Working in the media 1: options for doctors. *StudentBMJ.* 2004; **12**: 194–6.
9 Stillman P. Developing skills for the broadcast media. *BMJ Career Focus.* 1997; **314**: 2.
10 Leung WC. Career focus: combining medicine and law. *StudentBMJ.* 2000; **8**: 68–9.
11 Welch W, Kelly S. Premier league doctor. *StudentBMJ.* 2004; **12**: 286.
12 English B. Sports and exercise medicine. *StudentBMJ.* 2004; **12**: 282–3.

FURTHER READING

British Medical Association Medical Education Sub-Committee of the Board of Science. *Medical Specialties: the way forward*. London: British Medical Association; 2007.

Defence Deanery (www.gprecruitment.org.uk/deanery/defence.htm)

Defence Medical Services Department (www.dmsd.mod.uk)

Easton G. Working in the media 2: getting a foot in the door. *StudentBMJ*. 2004; **12**: 240–1.

Easton G. Working in the media 3: getting your message across. *StudentBMJ*. 2004; **12**: 284–5.

Kenny F. Creative medicine. *StudentBMJ*. 2006; **14**: 104–5.

www.bma.org.uk/employmentandcontracts/employmentcontracts/armed_forces/index.jsp (Section of the BMA website on working in the armed forces.)

Beasley R, Aldington S and Robinson G. From medical student to junior doctor: working outside the box. *StudentBMJ*. 2006; **14**: 238–9.

Sritharan K. A life on the ocean waves. *StudentBMJ*. 2006; **14**: 244–5.

20

What else can I do with a degree in medicine?

Just over a year after graduation, up to 20% of doctors have only a lukewarm desire to practise medicine, 4% have a weak desire and 2% regret becoming doctors.

This chapter is designed to give advice and make you aware of the options available to you should you decide that medicine is not for you.

Some medical students who manage to graduate choose not to work in medicine and may opt to pursue an alternative career. The knowledge that you gained whilst studying medicine may be invaluable in your new career.

After successfully completing a medical degree you will be the equivalent to any other graduate with a masters level degree. You can therefore attend graduate career fairs being an even match.[1] However, if you still wish to work in a medical related field you can think about medical journalism, medico-legal practice or working for the pharmaceutical industry. However, employers may prefer to appoint someone who has progressed further in their career and who has gained clinical experience by practising medicine. So if these careers do interest you it might be useful to stay in the NHS for a few years after qualifying to improve your chances in your chosen career outside mainstream medicine.

Medical graduates who go into careers that do not involve medicine are at a disadvantage compared with those who do. This is because they are only using their degree as currency, rather than as an advantage to their chosen career.[1] They may take a drop in salary as they change professions and may have decreased job security. Their pension rights may also be compromised.

The decision not to practise medicine or work in the medical field is hard. It should not be done for financial reasons, as you can end up earning less money,[2] having to retrain,[2] having lower job security and poorer pension structures by leaving the NHS.[2] If you think that you cannot deal with the demands placed on you by your medical career you should first step back and stop yourself from making a rash decision. There are ways of dealing with this pressure; for example:

- seeking career guidance
- adjusting your working conditions, (e.g. flexible working)
- addressing and amending, as appropriate, your work–life balance.

Alternatively, if you decide to take a break from medicine there may be incentive schemes to help you to return to the NHS at a later date. For example, the flexible returner scheme, which is part of the Flexible Careers Scheme, may still be available to you (*see* Chapter 13).

If you are considering leaving medical school or the medical profession, first take a look at Chapters 7 and 13. They might just make you change your mind!

The BMJ website contains articles organised by topic (http://careers.bmj.com/careers/advice/advice-overview.html). This is well worth a look at if you are considering using your medical degree away from the traditional career path as the topic headings include medical law, adventure medicine, improving working life, getting and changing jobs and, perhaps most relevant, leaving medicine. The latter contains articles about medics who have been on the traditional career path and experienced life away from medicine. These are well worth a read as they highlight the personal reasons why each clinician changed career path as well as the pros and cons of doing so.

Further information and advice can be found on the support4doctors website (www.support4doctors.org/advice.asp?catid=49&id=165) and through attending the Medical Success alternative career conferences (see the website for further information: www.medicalsuccess.net).

Name: Sonia Hutton-Taylor

Year of Graduation: 1983

Stage at which you left a traditional medical career path: after gaining FRCS and FRCOPhth

Career job: Started my own business in 1990: Medical Forum Career Management (www.medicalforum.com) – an independent medical human resources/medical education consultancy specialising in medical career guidance and planning.

Reasons for leaving traditional medical career path: Many and complex. Prefer being big cog in small wheel and total autonomy. Wasn't that fired up by surgery though could 'do' it and couldn't find anything else I wanted to do in medicine (although always interested in medicine and still am).

How do you use your medical degree in your current job: Every day I am talking to doctors, trusts and deaneries about medical careers. I did an occupational health (OH) diploma course two years ago (despite being out of medicine for 16 years – so did I ever leave?) because so much of my work overlaps OH. Although not a trained psychiatrist, my understanding of psychology, psychotherapy and mental illness is very useful.

Advice to students thinking about leaving traditional medical career path: If you have concerns or doubts, acknowledge them (even if most others you speak to don't – make finding someone who does a priority) and don't wait until you are completely burnt out, depressed or desperate to re-evaluate your career. The best career planning is done from a position of strength and energy. And don't think you are 'leaving' anything (wrong mindset) – think in terms of 'moving forward' (generally more constructive). There are literally dozens of careers one can do with a medical degree – its more to do with 'what you can/want to do' not what Dr Jo Bloggs 'medic' can do.

What would you do differently? I would have done more detailed careers researching between the ages of 22 and 25. I think that had I been able to access appropriate career guidance I would have found a niche within medicine like OH or healthcare MBA.

Are you happy with your career now? Very much indeed. It is always changing and never dull; it is creative and intellectually challenging.

Downsides: File phobia and accounts.

Do you regret doing medicine? Never.

Although most medical students can deal with the demands of an intensive course, some may find the pressure too intense. In every medical school there should be someone you can talk to about any problems you are having on your course. For instance, there may be a mentoring scheme in your medical school. More information on this can be found in Chapter 6. Those students who, in the first two years, feel that they no longer want to continue with medicine can sometimes transfer to another related course, such as pharmacology or biomedical sciences. Students who have managed to progress through the first year of clinical training may then decide that they do not want to continue studying medicine, and those who fail finals and re-sits may be eligible to be awarded a degree of biomedical science.

REFERENCES

1 Poole A. *What Are the Options to Medical Graduates Who Do Not Wish to Progress to the Preregistration House Officer Year?* BMJ Careers; 2004. Available at: http://careers.bmj.com/careers/advice/view-article.html?id=294 (accessed 15 January 2009).
2 Poole A. *What to Do with a Medical Degree if You Don't Want to Work in the NHS. Part 2: making the decision.* BMJ Careers; 2004. Available at http://careers.bmj.com/careers/advice/view-article.html?id=224 (accessed 15 January 2009).

FURTHER READING

Adams J. Is there life after medicine? *BMJ Career Focus.* 2003; **327**: 86.
Chambers R, Mohanna K and Field S. *Opportunities and Options in Medical Careers.* Oxford: Radcliffe Publishing; 2000.

Societies and organisations

This chapter introduces you to some of the societies and organisations that you may be in contact with throughout your medical career. The information has been written and/or approved by the organisations involved, which accounts for the slight variation in style and consistency of the writing; however, it ensures that information was correct at the time of print.

GENERAL MEDICAL COUNCIL

Main roles: accountability, discipline, registration, advice

General
Medical
Council

Regulating doctors
Ensuring good medical practice

The General Medical Council (GMC) has the legal power to protect, promote and maintain the health and safety of the community by ensuring proper standards in the practice of medicine.

The responsibilities of the GMC are listed below.

- Co-ordinates all stages and promotes high standards in medical association.
- Provisionally registers graduates of UK medical schools.
- Publishes guidance on general clinical training and its implementation.
- Grants full registration to doctors who gain the required competencies.
- Maintains a list and publishes a register of specialist doctors and, in the future, a list of GPs.
- Recognises qualifications awarded by EEA member states to EEA nationals.
- Regulates doctors.

The GMC website contains the guidelines mentioned above. These guidelines are useful and important in your education and practice throughout medical school. Other areas covered by the guidelines include consent of patients and conduct as a health professional (and medical student).

Website: www.gmc-uk.org

POSTGRADUATE MEDICAL EDUCATION AND TRAINING BOARD

Main roles: postgraduate medical education and training

PMETB

The Postgraduate Medical Education and Training Board (PMETB) is an independent regulatory body, responsible for promoting the development of postgraduate medical education across the UK.

It began operations on 30 September 2005, taking over the responsibilities of the Specialist Training Authority (STA) of the medical royal colleges and the Joint Committee on Postgraduate Training for General Practice (JCPTGP).

The vision that PMETB has set itself is to achieve excellence in postgraduate medical education, training, assessment and accreditation throughout the UK to improve the knowledge, skills and experience of doctors and the health and health-care of patients and the public.

The General and Specialist Medical Practice (Education, Training and Qualifications) Order 2003 (Statutory Instrument 2003 No. 1250) established the PMETB and defines its purpose – to develop postgraduate medical education and training.

PMETB's responsibilities at the time of print include:[1]
- certifying doctors for the GP and specialist registers
- prospective approval of all training posts that lead to the award of a CCT
- approving specialist training curricula and assessments
- setting the overarching principles under which selection into specialist training must operate.

However, there is a plan to merge the GMC and PMETB, creating a body called PGMET. At the time of print little more information is available, so look out for this and the remit for this new body.
Website: www.pmetb.org.uk

BRITISH MEDICAL ASSOCIATION
Main roles: advice, protection (of rights)

The British Medical Association (BMA) is the professional association for all UK doctors, and an independent trade union that is recognised by the government as a scientific 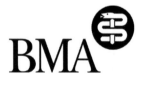 and educational body, with sole negotiating rights for doctors. As such, it represents doctors from all branches of medicine all over the UK, and has over 135 000 members, including over 16 000 student members.

The main aims of the BMA are to protect and support its members' professional interests and to negotiate with the government and NHS employers to bring about improvements in the profession and the NHS.

Student members receive a monthly copy of *StudentBMJ*, containing interesting political, lifestyle and educational articles, and opinions of medical students, accompanied by *Student BMA News*, featuring news, views and analysis.

For full details on the benefits of membership, visit the BMA website.
Website: www.bma.org.uk/_top/join_bma/index.jsp

MEDICAL DEFENCE UNION
Main roles: advice, protection

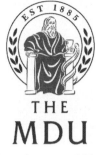

The Medical Defence Union (MDU) is a mutual, non-profit organisation, owned by its members – doctors, dentists and other healthcare professionals. Established in 1885, the MDU was the first medical defence organisation in the UK and provides members with advice and support throughout their studies and professional lives. As well as providing all the traditional discretionary benefits of a mutual, the MDU also provides its qualified members with the security of an insurance policy for indemnity up to £10 million.[2]

Other benefits of membership include:
- indemnity for Good Samaritan acts performed worldwide
- access to Freephone 24-hour advisory helpline
- discounted books, courses and educational services
- defence of professional reputations if clinical performance is called into question
- support in responding to patient complaints
- support with GMC or NHS disciplinary proceedings
- access to the MDU press office assisting with enquiries from the media
- access to case histories and advisory publications within the MDU website.

For further information about the benefits of MDU membership visit the website or contact the Membership Helpline on 0800 716376.
Website: www.the-mdu.com

MEDICAL AND DENTAL DEFENCE UNION OF SCOTLAND
Main roles: advice, protection, risk management

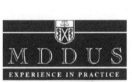

The Medical and Dental Defence Union of Scotland (MDDUS) is an independent UK-wide mutual indemnity organisation providing members with comprehensive indemnity and 24-hour advice and support.

Currently, the MDDUS has 25 000 members and is managed and governed by medical and dental practitioners. The aims of the MDDUS are to protect the professional interests of its members and to promote high standards of medical and dental practice.

Members have 24/7 access to clinically qualified medical advisers, uniquely experienced professionals with extensive understanding of the variety of situations encountered. This enables all situations to be managed sympathetically, effectively and in strict confidence.

Other services provided for members include:
- occurrence-based indemnity and support for legal action brought about by patients against general medical practitioners and specialists in private practice
- assistance with complaints

- professional advice and legal representation at GMC proceedings
- legal representation at fatal accident inquiries and coroner's inquests
- indemnity for assisting at emergencies and other occasions such as voluntary hospice work and worldwide Good Samaritan acts
- representation at disciplinary proceedings
- quarterly publication, *Summons*
- access to risk management advice in general medical practice
- advice and indemnity for the preparation of reports and expert opinions
- continued indemnity, after the member has ceased clinical practice, or left membership, for the period that they were in membership
- the option to put membership on hold if not working due to retirement, maternity leave or ill health – indemnity for Good Samaritan acts and *Summons* are still provided free of charge.

Membership costs depend upon specialty and length of practice, for advice on this you can contact the MDDUS. However, free membership is available to medical and dental students throughout the UK. Student membership provides benefits, including:
- free elective indemnity and a 'Guide to Electives'
- free advice booklets on topical medico-legal and practice issues
- quarterly publication, *Summons*, includes case studies and student pages
- discount on clinical textbooks from specified publishers, see the MDDUS website for further details
- involvement and sponsorship of student events, see the MDDUS website for further details.

Website: www.mddus.com

MEDICAL FORUM

Medical Forum is an independent 'career management facility' where doctors of all ages and backgrounds can explore their career concerns, situation, options and decisions. Medical Forum will help you to handle anything from a simple career choice through to more complex career dilemmas or crises. Medical Forum do not only offer career change advice but also, they work with consultants, GPs and trainees who are in post and not intending to change but who are facing career challenges. Not only this, if you are searching for new challenges, Medical Forum can help you to find them.

You can self refer to Medical Forum or you may be referred via deaneries, tutors or other medical organisations. For Medical Forum to work for you, you must be willing to learn and take charge of your career. They will not tell you what to do, but will help you to find this out for yourself.

If you would like to make full use of the services on offer from Medical Forum a charge will apply; however, you can decide which of the services may be of use to you for free by visiting website. The website provides free access to some services and

will allow you to obtain further information on all that is on offer.
Website: www.medicalforum.com

MEDICAL PROTECTION SOCIETY
Main roles: advice, protection

MEDICAL PROTECTION SOCIETY

The Medical Protection Society (MPS) prides itself on being the world's leading mutual medical protection organisation. It has the aim of providing help, in the form of protection and advice, to healthcare professionals with medico-legal problems that arise from their clinical practice.

A 24-hour telephone emergency advice line is offered. Services provided by the MPS are confidential. Specific and general situations that MPS members can ask for assistance with, include:

- clinical negligence claims
- complaints
- legal and ethical dilemmas
- GMC inquiries
- disciplinary procedures
- inquests and fatal accident inquiries
- police investigations relating to clinical practice.

In addition to assisting healthcare professionals with the above situations, the MPS also:

- has a role in risk management – working to promote safer practice
- lobbies to bring about a sensible regulatory environment
- can provide indemnity
- can provide legal representation
- can act as a spokesperson to the media.

The assistance offered by the MPS is given at the discretion of the MPS council, which consists mainly of medical and dental practitioners.

The MPS publishes a really useful journal, *Casebook*, as part of its work in promoting patient safety. *Casebook* is sent out to all MPS members and contains educational articles, letters and a really useful section that details previous cases where legal action has been sought. This latter section details the history of the case and what the outcome was. It then goes on to explain where errors occurred or what was good about the management. It is a really interesting tool that draws your attention to errors that have easily been made, but are potentially easy to avoid.
Website: www.mps.org.uk

HOWDEN MEDICAL INSURANCE SERVICES
Main roles: advice, protection

Complaints and allegations of negligence or poor

performance against medical practitioners are undoubtedly on the rise. On average a dentist or doctor is expected to receive one formal complaint for every two years they are in practice. Howden Medical Insurance Services (HMIS) is a new commercial company. However, the professional and medical risks division of Howden Insurance Brokers prides itself in having longstanding expertise in the field of medical malpractice. Doctors and dentists need to know that they have an indemnity insurance that is secure, reliable and supported by fully trained and experienced medico-legal experts. Backed by a consortium of London insurers, the HMIS team of medical, dental and claims specialists has launched a service tailored to meet the individual needs of dentists and doctors. HMIS provides cover for groups or individuals including: health authorities, medical associations, medical training colleges/universities, hospitals (public and private sector), clinics, medical practitioners (doctors, dentists, surgeons, chiropractors, osteopaths), other medical professionals (opticians, paramedics, pharmacists, nurses, chiropodists) and complementary medical practitioners (acupuncturists, homeopaths).

The cover HMIS offers may include:
- public and products liability
- protection against libel and slander
- cover for loss of documents
- supplementary legal expenses cover
- access to a range of helplines
- a range of 'run off' options.

Website: www.hmis.co.uk

WESLEYAN MEDICAL SICKNESS
Main roles: financial advice, income protection

Have you ever thought about what you would do if accident or illness prevented you from working and earning an income? The Medical Career Protector from Wesleyan Assurance Society is specifically designed for medical students and doctors. Exclusively provided through Wesleyan Medical Sickness, it is designed to protect your income should you suffer loss of earnings as a result of illness or accident. As a final-year medical student they can arrange cover for you free of charge, as they understand it is cover that you may not be able to afford. Then when you qualify as a doctor, under £30 per month will help to provide the cover you'll need in the early years of your career. In 2004 the Society paid over £36 million pounds in claims to doctors and dentists who were unable to work.

Wesleyan Medical Sickness has a dedicated team of student liaison managers covering medical schools across the UK who can provide information about and access to the cover. In addition they can provide sponsorship to school clubs, societies and events such as your Graduation Ball. They will also be co-ordinating your group photo – a tradition that Wesleyan Medical Sickness has upheld for over 30 years. Medical Sickness gives this photo to each and every final-year student, as a free gift from them, to remind you of your years at medical school.

Wesleyan Medical Sickness has been addressing the needs of medics since 1884 and is part of the Wesleyan Assurance Society, one of the oldest and financially strong mutual organisations in the UK. They also offer a wide range of insurance products for students, covering elective travel, motor and personal possessions.
Website: www.wesleyan.co.uk

MEDICAL WOMEN'S FEDERATION

Main roles: advice, representation of women in medicine

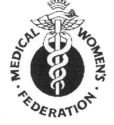

The Medical Women's Federation (MWF) is the largest and most influential body of women doctors in the UK.

The aims are to support women doctors in their personal and professional development, to remove gender barriers in the medical profession at all levels, and to improve the health of women and their families in society.

Annual student sponsorship:

- annual essay competition open to all medical students
- grants for medical student electives
- mature student grants for those with financial hardship.

They campaign on a number of issues, including flexible working and childcare, have representation on all important medical committees, input into major health policies and documents and, as part of the Medical Women's International Association, look at women's health issues globally.
Website: www.medicalwomensfederation.org.uk

PASTEST

Main roles: education, career support

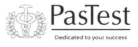

With over 30 years' experience of helping doctors and medical students pass their exams, PasTest provides high quality medical education. It provides a combination of books, courses, online revision, continuing professional development conferences and exhibitions. PasTest offers a complete career solution to medical students and doctors of all disciplines.
Website: www.pastest.co.uk

REFERENCES

1 Postgraduate Medical Education and Training Board. *Preparing Doctors for the Future: about PMETB*. Available at: www.pmetb.org.uk/fileadmin/user/Communications/Publications/Preparing_Doctors_for_the_future_About_PMETB.pdf (accessed 15 January 2009).
2 Subject to the terms and conditions of the Professional Indemnity Policy underwritten by Converium Insurance (UK) Ltd.
   MDU Services Limited (MDUSL) is authorised and regulated by the Financial Services Authority in respect of insurance mediation activities only. MDUSL is an agent for The Medical Defence Union Limited (the MDU). The MDU is not an insurance company. The benefits of membership of the MDU are all discretionary and are subject to the Memorandum and Articles of Association.

MDU Services Limited is registered in England 3957086 Registered Office: 230 Blackfriars Road London SE1 8PJ

22

Discrimination and how to avoid it

Discrimination is unacceptable. However, it is a real phenomenon occurring in medicine, as in other professions. It may not be apparent to everyone which groups or individuals are more vulnerable to discrimination or how this discrimination is manifested. This chapter highlights these points and suggests ways to avoid discrimination and, if it is already occurring, from where help can be sought.

Discrimination can occur as a result of illness, disease, disability, disfigurement, education, ethnic origin, religion, gender, age and sexual orientation. This list is not exhaustive, but it illustrates the diversity of traits that can lead to discrimination, and thus that discrimination could occur towards any of us. Discrimination may not be overt; all of us must be aware that we could each be a victim of discrimination. It is best to attempt to prevent discrimination from occurring in the first place as many people are reluctant to act against discrimination once it occurs, for fear of creating a detrimental effect on their career.

Negative effects of discrimination can include unhappiness, isolation and low self-esteem. In terms of careers, discrimination may result in limited and difficult career progression.

A career in medicine involves interaction with all members of the community from all walks of life. It is important that you understand how and why discrimination develops and is manifested so you will recognise it if you start to become a perpetrator.

Discrimination – or more accurately, preventing discrimination – is a major theme of the GMC, royal college and National Health Service (NHS) legislation and guidelines. The GMC's *Good Medical Practice*, *Tomorrow's Doctors* and *Duties of a Doctor* publications (*see* Chapter 11) each promote fair treatment of patients and colleagues. The NHS has set up flexible working, childcare, training and workforce retention initiatives to open up the opportunities of work to more people.[1] The BMA has insisted that bullying must stop and thus recommends zero tolerance. They have produced the report, *Bullying and Harassment of Doctors in the Workplace*, which can be found at www.bma.org.uk/employmentandcontracts/morale_motivation/bullying2006.jsp.

FORMS OF DISCRIMINATION

There are five basic types of discrimination.

Direct discrimination

Discrimination occurs directly as a result of a trait of a person (e.g. age, disability, religion, race, sex or sexual orientation). This discrimination would not occur should this trait not be present. Complainants alleging direct discrimination have to compare themselves with either an actual or hypothetical comparator to illustrate less favourable treatment.

Indirect discrimination

This occurs when a provision/criterion/practice is applied equally to all people but the effect of this is detrimental to a group of people because a considerably smaller proportion of people sharing a particular characteristic are able to comply.

Victimisation

Victimisation is unlawfully present when one person treats another less favourably than they treat others because the person has brought proceedings under a relevant piece of discrimination legislation, given evidence or information in connection with proceedings under a relevant piece of discrimination legislation, alleged that someone has contravened a relevant piece of discrimination legislation, or because the person believes that the victim has done or intends to do these things.

Harassment

This is said to occur when one person engages in unwanted conduct with another, based on a specific trait (e.g. sex, race, disability, etc.), which may violate that person's dignity or create an unpleasant environment for that person; for example intimidation, humiliation, offence.

Bullying

This is said to occur when power or status is misused to criticise, condemn and humiliate people, which may result in undermining their ability and/or confidence.

GENDER ISSUES

Gender is a dynamic cause of discrimination. Not only are proportions of men and women in medicine changing, but various specialties have differing male/female preponderances. Between 1990 and 2000, the total number of female hospital medical staff increased by 71%. In addition, the number of women entering medical school has doubled since the 1980s, with less than a 10% increase in male entrants over the same time.[2]

You may look at these figures and assume that women now dominate medicine, and that previous gender-based discrimination may be a thing of the past. However, women's progression in hospital medicine has been slower than expected and in 1998 only 20% of hospital consultants were women.[2]

Surgery has particularly low ratios of female to male consultants and registrars. Conversely, the greatest female to male ratios occur in clinical oncology, paediatrics, pathology, psychiatry and obstetrics and gynaecology.[2,3]

So what can be done with this information? First, do not let it put you off going into a specialty you are interested in. Discrimination can be so diverse that even if you are in a minority group it may not occur towards you if you are a female going into surgery. For instance, a 'Women in Surgical Training' initiative was established to encourage this by the Royal College of Surgeons and the Department of Health. Whether the apparent gender bias in various specialties is really due to discrimination or lifestyle choice is unclear. Be aware and ensure your chosen career path is not obscured by discrimination.

Transgender doctors may also present the potential for discrimination. Although many are happy and comfortable with their own situation, some may not be open about their sexuality for fear of others' negative reactions.

SEXUAL ORIENTATION

Many gay, lesbian and bisexual people are comfortable with their sexuality; however, fear of negative reactions from colleagues or patients can result in them not opening up to such people.[4] MacDonald stated that only half of clinical students believe homosexual activity can form part of an acceptable lifestyle.[5]

As a rule, when doctors are open about their sexuality, they have no problem. Discrimination in employment on the basis of sexual orientation is illegal – however, the possibility remains.[4]

ETHNIC ORIGIN

Ethnic minorities comprise 35% of hospital doctors.[2] However, this proportion is not uniform throughout grades. Only 20% of consultants are from an ethnic minority compared with 60% and 65% of associate specialists and staff grade doctors, respectively.[6] It is unclear how much of this inequality is a result of discrimination; however, if you are from a minority ethnic group, you should be vigilant to the potential of encountering unfair or discriminatory treatment. For example, medical schools have previously been criticised on the grounds of racism in the application process following the release of figures in 1999 that showed only 15% of ethnic minority applicants won places in medical schools compared to 55% of white applicants.[7] Similarly, research in 1997 revealed identical SHO applications were less likely to be shortlisted if the name was Asian rather than English.[8]

ILLNESS, DISEASE AND DISABILITY

Physical and mental illness can result in discrimination. In a world of 'caring professionals' the same professionals do not always appear as such when their own colleagues, or medical students, are involved. In particular, mental illness is a significant cause of discrimination.[5]

If you are disabled, your employers must not treat you less favourably as a result of your disability, unless action is justified. They must make reasonable adjustments to your working conditions or workplace to enable you to work more effectively/ easily. If your employer does not comply with these requirements they may be discriminating against you and you should research your rights, starting with the Disability Discrimination Act 1995 (DDA). It is important to realise the extent of the DDA. It covers disability caused by a wide range of conditions; for example, cancer,

HIV and facial disfigurement.

HOW TO AVOID DISCRIMINATING AGAINST PATIENTS AND COLLEAGUES

- Identify your own prejudices. We all have them and it is only by identifying them that we can attempt to prevent them from affecting our professional work and judgement.
- Remember that medical students and doctors with disabilities have already illustrated determination, intellectual ability and skills to get where they are – do not write them off.
- Understand your personality type (*see* Chapter 3) – the Myers-Briggs type indicator, a psychometric test used worldwide, involves a dimension that focuses on the way in which people make decisions. Grouping people by their decision-making styles, into 'thinkers' and 'feelers', creates groups, which may explain the development of bullying and/or discrimination. Thinkers are said to be exhilarated by conflict and may appear as tactless or abusive to feelers, despite the thinkers' intention being quite different. By understanding whether you are a thinker or a feeler, you may be able to manage situations more appropriately that may otherwise result in an act of discrimination.[9]
- Read articles about, or listen to, other people's experiences of discrimination and learn from them.
- Be aware of and avoid stereotyping people.
- Assess an individual's competencies and abilities based on their merits.
- Be aware that it is illegal to discriminate against people at work on the grounds of sex, sexual orientation, race, religion, disability, part-time working or being, or not being, a member of a trades union.
- Realise that people with chronic conditions are often the experts of their own medical problems and lifestyle requirements; if you are unsure of anything just ask.

HOW TO AVOID BEING DISCRIMINATED AGAINST

Giving generic tips on how to avoid discrimination directed at you is difficult due to the diversity of traits that result in discrimination. The following list has been written to be interpreted in a 'where applicable' fashion.

- Be open and honest with yourself and your colleagues,[10] you do not have to tell everyone in every case, but make sure you are honest with those to whom it legally and ethically matters.
- Maintain your health at the best that you can while avoiding excessive time off work as time off work can lead to time out of training and thus a deficiency of skills or knowledge:
  - try and keep doctors' appointments out of your working hours if possible
  - be compliant with your medication and treatment
  - generally maintain good health by eating regularly and taking regular breaks, especially if you need more than others, due to illness.
- Identify problems you have which may lead to discrimination and think about

ways of overcoming or adapting to these problems;[10] this may include the use of aids, gadgets or alterations to the workplace.

- Seek help from relevant people or organisations, which may include:
  - colleagues
  - employers – they are liable for acts of discrimination carried out by their employees, regardless of knowledge or approval; employers are also liable if considered to have failed to prevent employees suffering discrimination in the workplace, therefore, it is in your employer's interest to take a part in preventing discrimination
  - postgraduate deanery
  - occupational health department
  - support groups – limited details can be found in Appendix 1
  - 'Access to Work' – a government scheme run through local job centre plus offices which conducts workplace assessments and can provide advice on and funding for (in certain circumstances) extra equipment or costs incurred which may be needed for your employment
  - BMJ Careers chronic illness matching scheme
  - Association for Disabled Professionals – provides advice and runs a network support scheme which matches professionals with similar disabilities and jobs to provide support for each other
  - Workstep – will put you in touch with a disability employment adviser and provides job support to disabled employees
  - Equality and Human Rights Commission – provides advice, support and legal information to help ensure the rights of the groups represented are protected.
- Know your rights and do not be forced into decisions you will regret (e.g. lower posts, retirement) – certain documents, acts and regulations have been produced and organisations exist to assist with legal issues:
  - The Disability Discrimination Act 1995 and 2005 – produced to ensure employers fulfil their responsibilities to you and provide additional resources to assist you in performing your job
  - The Employment Equality (age) Regulations 2006 – address discrimination on the grounds of age
  - The Employment Equality (religion or belief) Regulations 2003 – cover discrimination on the grounds of religion
  - The Employment Equality (sexual orientation) Regulations 2003 – it is illegal to discriminate against people at work on the basis of their sexual orientation
  - Prevention of Less Favourable Treatment Regulations 2000 – produced to prevent discrimination of part-time workers, ensuring equal pay, inclusion in appropriate training, adequate holiday entitlement, availability of career break schemes (e.g. maternity leave) and fair consideration at times of redundancy
  - Race Relations Act 1976 (Amendment) Regulations 2003

■ Sex Discrimination Act 1975 – it is illegal to discriminate against people at work on the basis of their sex.

Lastly, it is important that you ensure you maintain good social relationships to provide a good source of support should these preventative measures fail.

WHAT YOU CAN DO IF DISCRIMINATION OCCURS

Your instinct may be not to act. However, you should think carefully before doing this. If you feel you are being discriminated against, the chances are some of your colleagues may be as well. This decision should be made relatively quickly, as you only have three months minus one day from the date of the act of discrimination to submit an application to an employment tribunal.[1]

If you make a complaint of discrimination your employer is expected to deal with this promptly, objectively, thoroughly and with due regard to confidentiality. They are duty bound to do this, not only for your benefit but for their own. The employer's commitment to equal opportunities will be judged on the basis of how they deal with situations such as this. If your employer does not deal with your complaint appropriately their actions may be interpreted as approval of the discrimination.[1]

In order to make a good case for discrimination, bullying or harassment, you will need to collect evidence and record details of what has been happening. Keeping a diary, which logs the events and any witnesses, can be helpful. In addition, any letters, e-mails or other permanent items of communication should be kept.[11]

The BMA will take on cases of members only if their associated lawyers decide they have at least a 50% chance of winning. For those whose cases are not taken on, the BMA also offers their members a counselling line for support.[12]

Once you have taken action for alleged discrimination, the case will be assessed for its suitability to be resolved informally. However, it is also recommended that you submit an application to an employment tribunal immediately due to tight time restrictions. If your case is not deemed suitable for informal resolution it will be passed through your employer's procedure for dealing with complaints of alleged discrimination. Severe cases may require resolution under your employer's disciplinary policy.[1]

REFERENCES

1 British Medical Association. *Dealing with Discrimination: guidelines for BMA members*. London: British Medical Association; 2004.

2 Jackson C, Ball JE, Hirsh W, *et al*. *Informing Choices: the need for career advice in medical training*. Cambridge: National Institute for Careers Education Counselling; 2003.

3 Allen I. Women doctors and their careers: what now? *BMJ*. 2005; **331**: 569–72.

4 Gay and Lesbian Association of Doctors and Dentists, 2005. Available at: www.gladd.co.uk (accessed 15 January 2009).

5 MacDonald R. Discrimination in medicine. *BMJ*. 2002; **324**: 1112.

6 Cooke L, Halford S and Leonard P. *Racism in the Medical Profession: the experience of UK graduates*. British Medical Association: London; 2003.

7 British Medical Association Central Consultants and Specialists Committee. *Tackling Racism in Medical Careers: the role of consultants – policy paper*. British Medical Association: London; 2005. Available at: www.bma.org/ap.nsf/Content/TacklingRacisminMedicalCareers (accessed 15 January 2009).

8 Esmail A and Everington S. Asian doctors are still being discriminated against. *BMJ*. 1997; **314**: 1619.

9 Paice E and Firth-Cozens J. Who's a bully then? *BMJ Career Focus*. 2003; **326**: 127.

10 Stiff RE. Life as a visually impaired doctor. *BMJ Career Focus*. 2004; **329**: 15–16.

11 British Medical Association Career Focus. *Overseas Doctors: sink or swim*. London: British Medical Association; 2004.

12 Cohen D and Hebert K. Equality and diversity in the workplace. *BMJ Career Focus*. 2004; **329**: 116–17.

FURTHER READING

British Medical Association. *Sexual Orientation in the Workplace*. London: British Medical Association; 2005.

Gay and Lesbian Association of Doctors and Dentists. *Improving Working Lives: guidelines on dignity at work for lesbian and gay doctors and dentists, medical and dental students*; 2004. Available at: www.gladd.org.uk

Appendix 1

RESOURCES

Chapter 1: Introduction

BMJ Careers: www.bmjcareers.com
Foundation Programme: www.foundationprogramme.nhs.uk
Making sense of your medical career: www.yourmedicalcareer.com
Modernising Medical Careers: www.mmc.nhs.uk

Chapter 2: Experiences of others

GP recruitment: www.gprecruitment.org.uk (Includes information on GP careers, day in the life of a GP, qualities of a good GP, vacancies, information and links to all UK deanery websites)
NHS Careers: www.nhscareers.nhs.uk/medical.shtml
West Midlands Workforce Deanery podcasts: www.westmidlands.nhs.uk/cms/ WorkforceDeanery/MedicalCareers/SpecialtyTrainee/SpecialtyInformation/ tabid/503/Default.aspx

Chapter 3: Career development toolkit

Modernising Medical Careers: www.mmc.nhs.uk
NHS professionals: www.nhsprofessionals.nhs.uk

Chapter 4: Preparation for future jobs

Medical Forum www.medicalforum.com
Careers Group www.careers.lon.ac.uk [Includes a poor résumé and the same information presented well]
Doctors' Supportline: www.dsn.org.uk
    Tel: 087 0765 0001
    38 Harwood Road, London, SW6 4PH
Doctors' Support Network: www.dsn.org.uk
    Tel: 087 0321 0642
    PO Box 360, Stevenage, SG1 9AS
Doctors' Support Network Wales and Southwest:
    Tel: 087 0321 0642 or
    5 Borage Close, Pontprennaeu, Cardiff, CF23 8SJ

GP recruitment: www.gprecruitment.org.uk
Jobscore: http://doctors.jobscore.co.uk
Medical interviews: www.medical-interviews.co.uk
Modernising Medical Careers: www.mmc.nhs.uk

Chapter 5: Career support, advisers and fairs

BMJ Careers: http://careers.bmj.com
BMJ Careers Fairs: http://careersfair.bmj.com
Medical Forum www.medicalforum.com
Modernising Medical Careers: www.mmc.nhs.uk

Chapter 6: Mentors and educational supervisors

Academy of Medical Sciences Mentoring Scheme for academic careers: www.acmedsci.ac.uk/

Chapter 7: What is good about a career in medicine?

NHS careers: www.nhscareers.nhs.uk

Chapter 8: Medical career pathways

Foundation Programme: www.foundationprogramme.nhs.uk
Modernising Medical Careers: www.mmc.nhs.uk

Chapter 9: The Foundation Programme

Foundation Programme: www.foundationprogramme.nhs.uk
Jobscore: http://doctors.jobscore.co.uk/login.php?redirectTo=index.php

Chapter 10: Broadening your clinical experience

Community Service Volunteers: www.csv.org.uk
Concordia: www.concordia-iye.org.uk
Department of Health: www.dh.gov.uk (A home of publications and policies)
Medics Travel: www.medicstravel.co.uk
MedSin: www.medsin.org
National Institute of Clinical Excellence: www.nice.org.uk (A home of publications and policies)
National Library for Health: www.library.nhs.uk
National Travel Health Network and Centre: www.nathnac.org/travel/index.htm
NHS Access to Healthcare Abroad: www.nhs.uk/Healthcareabroad/Pages/Health careabroad.aspx (information on moving abroad, travelling abroad, travel health and country-by-country information)
Voluntary Services Overseas: www.vso.org.uk
Work the World: www.worktheworld.co.uk

Chapter 11: Application to Foundation Programme posts

Foundation Programme: www.foundationprogramme.nhs.uk

General Medical Council: www.gmc-uk.org
Scottish Foundation Allocation Scheme: www.nes.scot.nhs.uk/sfas/

Chapter 13: Postgraduate working conditions and pay

British Medical Association: www.bma.org.uk
NHS Pensions agency: www.nhsbsa.nhs.uk/pensions

Chapter 14: Specialty Training

GP recruitment: www.gprecruitment.org.uk
Jobscore: http://doctors.jobscore.co.uk/login.php?redirectTo=index.php
Modernising Medical Careers competition ratios: www.mmc.nhs.uk/default.aspx?
    page=348
West Midlands Workforce Deanery podcasts: www.westmidlands.nhs.uk/cms/
    WorkforceDeanery/MedicalCareers/SpecialtyTrainee/SpecialtyInformation/
    tabid/503/Default.aspx

Chapter 15: Specialty profiles

NHS Careers: www.nhscareers.nhs.uk/medical.shtml
West Midlands Workforce Deanery specialty pages: www.westmidlands.nhs.uk/
    cms/WorkforceDeanery/MedicalCareers/SpecialtyTrainee/SpecialtyInformation/
    tabid/503/Default.aspx

Chapter 16: Academic medicine: incorporating research and medical education into your career

Academy of Medical Sciences: www.acmedsci.ac.uk
Association for the Study of Medical Education: www.asme.org.uk
Foundation Programme academic pages: www.foundationprogramme.nhs.uk/
    pages/academic-programmes
Medical Research Council: www.mrc.ac.uk
National Institute for Health Research: www.nihr.ac.uk
NIHR Coordinating Centre for Research Capacity Development: www.nccrcd.
    nhs.uk
Society of Academic Foundation Trainees: http://saftuk.org/portal/
UK Clinical Research Collaboration: www.ukcrc.org
Wellcome Trust: www.wellcome.ac.uk

Chapter 17: GPs with special interests

Association of Practitioners with Special Interests http://apwsi.co.uk/
Primary Care Contracting website section on Practitioners with Special Interests
    www.pcc.nhs.uk/173.php

Chapter 18: Working abroad

Australian Government Department of Immigration and Citizenship: www.immi.
    gov.au [Information on visas and immigration]

Australian High Commission: www.australia.org.uk [For visas needed to work in Australia]

Australian Medical Council: www.amc.org.au

British Foreign and Commonwealth Office: www.fco.gov.uk/en/

Education Commission for Foreign Medical Graduates: www.ecfmg.org [USA site]

International Medical Recruitment: www.imrmedical.com [Medical jobs in Australia and New Zealand]

Medics Travel: www.medicstravel.com

Medrecruit: www.medrecruit.com [Job placements for doctors in Australia and New Zealand]

United States Medical Licensing Exam: www.usmle.org

Work the World: www.worktheworld.co.uk [Provider of professionally organised healthcare student placements in Africa and Asia]

Chapter 19: Diverse medical careers

British Association of Sport and Exercise Medicine: www.basem.co.uk

British Institute of Musculoskeletal Medicine: www.bimm.org.uk

United Kingdom Association of Doctors in Sport: www.ukadis.org

Chapter 20: What else can I do with a degree in medicine?

BMJ articles by topic: http://careers.bmj.com/careers/advice/advice-overview.html

Medical Forum: www.medicalforum.com

Medical Success: www.medicalsuccess.net

Support 4 Doctors: www.support4doctors.org/advice.asp?catid=49&id=165

Chapter 21: Societies and organisations

British Medical Association: www.bma.org.uk
Tel: 020 7387 4499
BMA House, Tavistock Square, London, WC1H 9JP

General Medical Council: www.gmc-uk.org
Tel: 0845 357 3456
Regent's Place, 350 Euston Road, London NW1 3JN

Howden Medical Insurance Services: www.hmis.co.uk
Tel: 020 7623 3806
Howden Insurance Brokers, Bevis Marks House, Bevis Marks, London, EC3A 7NE

Medical Defence Union: www.the-mdu.com

Medical and Dental Defence Union of Scotland: www.mddus.com
Tel: 0141 221 5858
Mackintosh House, 120 Blythswood Street, Glasgow, G2 4EA

Medical Forum: www.medicalforum.com
Tel: 0208 332 1234
Medical Forum River Cottage, Overton, Hants, RG25 3EB

Medical Insurance Agency: www.towergate.co.uk
   Tel: 01438 739739
   MIA, Kings Court, London Road, Stevenage, Herts, SG1 2GA
Medical Protection Society: www.mps.org.uk
   Tel: 0845 605 4000
   Medical Protection Society, Granary Wharf House, Leeds, LS11 5PY
Medical Sickness: www.medical-sickness.co.uk/
   Tel: 0808 100 1884
Wesleyan Assurance Society, Colmore Circus, Birmingham, B4 6AR
Medical Women's Federation: www.medicalwomensfederation.org.uk
   Tel: 020 7387 7765
   Tavistock House North, Tavistock Square, London, WC1H 9HX
Medical Women's International Association: www.mwia.net/
PasTest: www.pastest.co.uk
   Tel: 0156 5752 000
   PasTest, Egerton Court, Parkgate Estate, Knutsford, Cheshire, WA16 8DX
Postgraduate Medical Education and Training Board: www.pmetb.org.uk
   Tel: 020 7160 6100
   PMETB, Hercules House, Hercules Road, London, SE1 7DU

Chapter 22: Discrimination and how to avoid it

Abilitynet: www.abilitynet.co.uk
Access to work: www.direct.gov.uk/en/DisabledPeople/Employmentsupport/Work
   SchemesAndProgrammes/DG_4000347
Advisory, Conciliation and Arbitration Service (ACAS): www.acas.org.uk/
Association of Disabled Professionals: www.adp.org.uk
British Medical Association: www.bma.org.uk
Citizens Advice Bureau: www.nacab.org.uk/
Department for Business Enterprise and Regulatory Reform: www.berr.gov.uk
Disability Discrimination Act: www.direct.gov.uk/en/DisabledPeople/RightsAnd
   Obligations/DisabilityRights/DG_4001068
Doctors' Supportline: www.dsn.org.uk
Doctors' Support Network: www.dsn.org.uk
Doctors' Support Network Wales and Southwest: Tel: 087 0321 0642
Employment Law: www.compactlaw.co.uk/monster/empf30.html
Equality and human rights commission: www.equalityhumanrights.com
Equality commission for Northern Ireland: www.equalityni.org
Gay and Lesbian Association for Doctors and Dentist (GLADD): www.gladd.org.
   uk
Medical Council on Alcohol: www.medicouncilalcol.demon.co.uk
SKILL: national bureau for students with disabilities: www.skill.org.uk
Workstep: www.direct.gov.uk/en/DisabledPeople/Employmentsupport/Work
   SchemesAndProgrammes/DG_4001973

Appendix 2

CURRENT CAREER INTERESTS

Date

What type of career interests you at the moment?

Which areas of future career possibilities do not interest you?

Strengths

What are your strengths?

Weaknesses

What are your weaknesses?

Opportunities

What opportunities are available to help you pursue your career of interest?

Threats

What obstacles to your future career do you face?

What, if anything, can you do to overcome your weaknesses?

What is your ideal work–life balance?

What are your career aspirations?

Looking at the answers to the above, and at the appropriate specialty profile within this book, comment on your suitability to your career of interest.

What expectations, questions or concerns do you have at this stage about your career?

Photocopy this page for your own use

Appendix 3

USING CLINICAL ATTACHMENTS TO FURTHER CAREER DEVELOPMENT DECISIONS

Attachment

Date

Which aspects of this attachment did you enjoy?

Which aspects of this attachment did you not enjoy?

What type of experiences were you exposed to?

What did you learn about yourself during this attachment?

What feedback did you receive?

What strengths do you think are required for a career within this specialty?

Which aspects of this attachment would you like to do more of in the future?

Would you consider the area of your attachment for your future career? (State reasons)

Photocopy this page for your own use

Appendix 4

REFLECTION FOR BEGINNERS

Complete this table at the end of each week. Look back over the week's events and answer each question as fully as possible.

What is the best thing that happened this week? What happened? Where were you? Why did it happen? What can you do to make it/something similar to happen again? What have you learned?	
What is the worst thing that happened this week? What happened? Where were you? Why did it happen? What can you do to prevent it/something similar happening again? What have you learned?	
What was the most rewarding thing that happened this week? What happened? Where were you? Why did it happen? What can you do to make it/something similar happen again? What have you learned?	
What was the least rewarding thing that happened this week? What happened? Where were you? Why did it happen? What can you do to prevent it/something similar happening again? What have you learned?	

Appendix 5

REFLECTION FOR EVERYBODY

Complete this table every time something significant, memorable, good or bad happens. You can do this daily, multiple times a day or once a week. The more you do it the better you will know yourself and your capabilities.

Date:	
Give a brief overview of the event, occurrence or situation that you will reflect upon. What happened? Where were you? Who was involved?	
Who was affected by this event, occurrence or situation and how was each person/ group of people affected?	
What issues have arisen for you as a result of this event, occurrence or situation? Perhaps your knowledge is lacking? Maybe you were affected emotionally? Write down everything.	
What actions will you take as a result of this event, occurrence or situation? Do you need to speak to someone? Do you need to seek advice from a medical defence organisation? Do you need to change the way you approach certain situations?	
What do you need to know/ask about as a result of this event, occurrence or situation? Include a list of possible sources of advice or information.	
What was the final outcome for you, whoever was involved and/or the further actions that resulted from this event, occurrence or situation?	

Appendix 6

CONTACT DETAILS FOR THE ROYAL COLLEGES

Academy of Medical Royal Colleges 1 Wimpole Street, London W1G 0AE (+44 (0)20 740 82244; www.aomrc.org.uk).

Royal College of Anaesthetists 48/49 Russell Square, London WC1B 4JP (+44 (0)20 790 87300; www.rcoa.ac.uk).

Royal College of General Practitioners 14 Princes Gate, Hyde Park, London SW7 1PU (+44 (0)20 758 13232; www.rcgp.org.uk).

Royal College of General Practitioners Northern Ireland Building 4, Ground Floor, Cromac Place, Ormeau Road, Belfast BT7 2JB (+44 (0)289 023 0055; www.rcgp-ni.org.uk).

Royal College of General Practitioners Scotland 25 Queen Street, Edinburgh EH2 1JX (+44 (0)131 260 6800; www.rcgp-scotland.org.uk).

Royal College of General Practitioners Wales Regus House, Falcon Drive, Cardiff Bay, Cardiff CF10 4RU (+44 (0)292 050 4604; www.rcgp.wales.nhs.uk).

Royal College of Obstetricians and Gynaecologists 27 Sussex Place, London NW1 4RG (+44 (0)20 777 26200; www.rcog.org.uk).

Royal College of Ophthalmologists 17 Cornwall Terrace, London NW1 4QW (+44 (0)20 793 50702; www.rcophth.ac.uk).

Royal College of Paediatrics and Child Health 50 Hallam Street, London W1N 6DE (+44 (0)20 730 75600; www.rcpch.ac.uk).

Royal College of Pathologists 2 Carlton House Terrace, London SW1Y 5AF (+44 (0)20 745 16700; www.rcpath.org).

Royal College of Physicians 11 St Andrew's Place, Regent's Park, London NW1 4LE (+44 (0)20 793 51174; www.rcplondon.ac.uk).

Royal College of Physicians of Edinburgh 9 Queen Street, Edinburgh EH2 1JQ (+44 (0)131 225 7324; www.rcpe.ac.uk).

Royal College of Physicians and Surgeons of Glasgow 232–42 St Vincent Street, Glasgow G2 5RJ (+44 (0)141 221 6072; www.rcpsglasg.ac.uk).

Royal College of Psychiatrists 17 Belgrave Square, London SW1X 8PG (+44 (0)20 723 52351; www.rcpsych.ac.uk).

Royal College of Psychiatrists Northern Irish Division Forsyth Business Centre, 2–14 East Bridge Street, Belfast BT1 3MQ (+44 (0)289 092 3763; www.rcpsych.ac.uk/college/division/northern ireland.asp).

Royal College of Psychiatrists Scottish Division 12 Queen Street, Edinburgh EH2 1JE (+44 (0)131 220 2915; www.rcpsych.ac.uk/college/division/scot.asp).

Royal College of Psychiatrists Welsh Division Baltic House, Mount Stuart Square, Cardiff CF10 5FH (+44 (0)292 048 9006; www.rcpsych.ac.uk/college/ division/welsh.asp).

Royal College of Radiologists 38 Portland Place, London W1N 3DG (+44 (0)20 763 64432; www. rcr.ac.uk).

Royal College of Surgeons of England 25–43 Lincoln's Inn Fields, London WC2A 3PN (+44 (0)20 740 53474; www.rcseng.ac.uk).

Royal College of Surgeons of Edinburgh Nicolson Street, Edinburgh EH89DW (+44 (0)131 527 1600; www.rcsed.ac.uk). Appendix 4 151

Appendix 7

MEDICAL SCHOOLS IN THE UK

All contact details are correct at the time of print. The medical schools listed below run various medical degrees; to get more detailed information, e-mail addresses and information on each university, please visit the websites listed below. The website addresses in brackets are for the medical schools.

Aberdeen – School of Medicine, University of Aberdeen, Polwarth Building, Foresterhill, Aberdeen AB25 2ZD +44 (0)122 455 3015/4975 www.abdn.ac.uk (www.abdn.ac.uk/medicine)

Belfast – Queen's University, Whitla Medical Building, 97 Lisburn Road, Belfast BT9 7BL +44 (0)289 033 5778 www.qub.ac.uk (www.qub.ac.uk/cm)

Birmingham – The University of Birmingham, Edgbaston, Birmingham B15 2TT +44 (0)121 414 6888/3687 www.bham.ac.uk (www.medicine.bham.ac.uk)

Brighton – Brighton and Sussex Medical School, BSMS Teaching Building, University of Sussex, Brighton BN1 9PX +44 (0)127 364 4644 www.bsms.ac.uk (www.bsms.ac.uk)

Bristol – Faculty of Medicine and Dentistry, 69 St Michael's Hill, Bristol BS1 8DZ +44 (0)117 928 7679 www.bristol.ac.uk (www.medici.bris.ac.uk)

Cambridge – University of Cambridge, School of Clinical Medicine, Addenbrooke's Hospital, Hills Road, Cambridge CB2 2SP +44 (0)122 333 6700 www.cam.ac.uk (www.medschl.cam.ac.uk)

Cardiff – University of Wales, School of Medicine Registry, University of Wales College of Medicine, Heath Park, Cardiff CG14 4XN +44 (0)292 074 2027/3436 www.cardiff.ac.uk (www.cardiff.ac.uk/medicine)

Dundee – Faculty of Medicine, Dentistry and Nursing, University of Dundee, Level 10, Ninewells Hospital and Medical School, Dundee DD1 9YS +44 (0)138 263 2763 www.dundee.ac.uk (www.dundee.ac.uk/medical school)

Durham – Stockton, University of Durham, Queen's Campus Stockton, University Boulevard, Stockton-on-Tees TS17 6BH +44 (0)191 334 0048 www.dur.ac.uk (www.dur.ac.uk/phase1.medicine)

Edinburgh – College of Medicine and Veterinary Medicine, The University of Edinburgh, The Queen's Medical Research Institute, 47 Little France Crescent, Edinburgh EH16 4TJ +44 (0)131 242 9300 www.ed.ac.uk (www.mvm.ed. ac.uk)

Glasgow – Faculty of Medicine, Wolfson Medical School Building, University Avenue, University of Glasgow G12 8QQ +44 (0)141 330 5921 www.gla.ac.uk (www.gla.ac.uk/departments/medicine royal./home.htm)

Hull – The University of Hull, Hull HU6 7RX +44 (0)148 246 4705 (www.hyms.ac.uk)

Keele – School of Medicine, Keele University, Keele ST5 5BG +44 (0)178 258 3642/3632 www.keele.ac.uk (www.keele.ac.uk/depts/ms)

Leeds – Faculty of Medicine and Health, Worsley Building, University of Leeds, Leeds LS2 9JT +44 (0)113 343 7194 www.leeds.ac.uk (www.leeds.ac.uk/ medicine/index.html)

Leicester – University of Leicester, Medical School, University Road, Leicester LE1 7RH +44 (0)116 252 5281 www.le.ac.uk (www.le.ac.uk/sm/le)

Liverpool – University of Liverpool, Faculty of Medicine, Duncan Building, Daulby Street, Liverpool L69 3GA +44 (0)151 706 4261 www.liv.ac.uk (www.liv.ac.uk/medicine)

London – Barts and The London, Queen Mary University of London, Turner Street, London E1 2AD +44 (0)20 737 77611 www.qmul.ac.uk (www.mds.qmw.ac.uk)

London – King's College, King's College London School of Medicine, First Floor, Hodgkin Building, Guys Campus, London SE1 9RT +44 (0)20 783 65454 www.klc.ac.uk (www.kcl.ac.uk/teares/ gktvc)

London – Imperial College, Imperial College School of Medicine, South Kensington Campus, London SW7 2AZ +44 (0)20 759 48800 www.imperial.ac.uk (www1.imperial.ac.uk/medicine/default/ html)

London – Royal Free and University College, University College London, Gower Street, London WC1E 6BT +44 (0)20 767 97050 www.ucl.ac.uk (www. ucl.ac.uk/medicalschool)

London – St George's, St George's Hospital Medical School, Cranmer Terrace, London SW17 0RE +44 (0)20 867 29944 www.sgul.ac.uk

Manchester – The University of Manchester, Oxford Road, Manchester M13 9PL +44 (0)161 275 2077 www.manchester.ac.uk (www.medicine.manchester. ac.uk)

Newcastle upon Tyne – University of Newcastle upon Tyne, 10 Kensington Terrace, Newcastle upon Tyne NE1 7RU +44 (0)191 222 5594 www.ncl.ac.uk (www.medical.faculty.ncl.ac.uk)

Norwich – University of East Anglia, School of Medicine, Norwich NR4 7TJ +44 (0)160 345 6161 www.uea.ac.uk (www.med.uea.ac.uk)

Nottingham – Faculty of Medicine and Health Sciences, University of Nottingham Medical School, Queen's Medical Centre, Nottingham NG7 2UH +44 (0)115 970 9379 www.nottingham.ac.uk (www.nottingham.ac.uk/mhs)

Oxford – The Medical Sciences Office, University of Oxford, The John Radcliffe Hospital, Oxford OX3 9DU +44 (0)186 522 1689 www.ox.ac.uk (www. medsci.ox.ac.uk)

Peninsula Medical School – Peninsula Medical School, John Bull Building, Research Way, Plymouth PL6 8BU +44 (0)175 243 7444 www.pms.ac.uk (www.pms.ac.uk/pms)

Sheffield – School of Medicine and Biomedical Sciences, University of Sheffield, Beech Hill Road, Sheffield S10 2RX +44 (0)114 271 3349 www.sheffield.ac.uk (www.shef.ac.uk/medicine)

Southampton – School of Medicine, Southampton General Hospital, Tremona Road, Southampton SO16 6yd +44 (0)238 079 6586 www.soton.ac.uk (www. som.soton.ac.uk)

St Andrews – The University of St Andrews, 79 North Street, St Andrews KY16 9AJ +44 (0)133 446 2150/3502 www.st-and.ac.uk (http://medicine.stand. ac.uk)

Swansea – University of Wales, School of Medicine, Grove Building, University of Wales Swansea, Singleton Park, Swansea SA2 8PP +44 (0)179 251 3400 www2.swan.ac.uk (www.medicine.swan. ac.uk)

Warwick – Warwick Medical School, The University of Warwick, Coventry CV4 7AL +44 (0)247 652 3523 www.warwick.ac.uk (www2.warwick.ac.uk/fac/ med/)

York – The University of York, Heslington, York YO10 5DD +44 (0)190 432 1969 (www.hyms. ac.uk)

Index

academic clinical fellowships (ACF) 56, 102, 126–7, 130
academic medicine 19, 71, 126–9, 166
Academy of Medical Royal Colleges 173
'Access to Work' scheme 161
accident and emergency (A&E) *see also* emergency medicine
  career pathway 4–5
  experience in 64, 65, 110
  personality toolkit 19
  premier league doctor 144
  ship's doctor 143
  specialty profile 107–8
acute medicine 14, 54, 55, 56, 61, 62, 108, 109, 110, 111
Africa 138
age discrimination 161
age-related medicine (geriatrics) 13, 108–9, 143
aid agencies 140
Air Force careers 141–2
Alberta, Canada website 139–40
alcohol 26, 95, 97, 113
Alternative Career Paths for Doctors career fair 40
alternative careers 40, 146–8, 167
anaesthetics 55, 109–10, 136
annual leave 90, 93, 142
Annual Review of Competence Progression 104
applications *see* job applications
appraisals 60, 62, 76
Army careers 141–2
Aspiring to Excellence (Tooke report) 52–3, 54–5, 56, 100, 127
Association for Disabled Professionals 161
Association for Graduate Careers Advisory Services (AGCAS) 35
Association for the Study of Medical Education (ASME) 130
asylum seekers 44, 134
audits, clinical 51, 100, 101
Australia 138, 139, 166
Australian Medical Council exams 137

BAMMbino 55
bisexual doctors 159, 161
BMJ see *British Medical Journal*
British Association for Sexual Health and HIV 117
British Cardiovascular Society 111

British Geriatric Society 109
British Medical Association 13
  A Career in Academic Medicine 126
  Cohort Study of 2006 Medical Graduates 1, 13, 60
  discrimination 162
  elective funding information 69
  Junior Doctors' Handbook 91, 92
  Medical Specialties 99
  mentoring 41
  overview 150
  pay banding calculators 90
  pensions information 92
  working abroad, guidance 139, 140
British Medical Journal (BMJ) 9, 101
  BMJ Career Focus 31
  BMJ Careers 35, 39–40, 100, 101, 147, 161
  Student BMJ 10, 16, 150
British Orthopaedic Society 121
British Society for Rheumatology 125
British Society of Gastroenterologists 114
bullying 157, 158, 160, 162
Bullying and Harassment of Doctors in the Workplace 157

Canada 69, 139–40
cardiology 110–11, 134, 143
career advice 32–3, 34–5, 36–7, 146, 152–3
career advisers 1, 36–7, 165
career decisions, components of 8–9
career development toolkit
  competition ratios 11–13, 14, 80
  interactive resources 10–11, 13–20, 34, 169, 170
  managing career development 8–9
  mentoring 42
  personality type 13–19, 34
  resources 164
career education 42–3
career fairs, forums and events 33, 37–40, 100, 146, 165
A Career in Academic Medicine 126
career management 42
Career Management 32, 34–5, 36
career pathways 4–7, 48, 50, 51, 54–6, 165 *see also* training
career support 1, 31–6, 48, 52, 76, 99, 152–3, 155, 164–5

careers, alternative 40, 146–8, 167
case-based discussion 59
Casebook 9, 153
Certificate of Completion of Training (CCT) 50, 55, 100, 104, 105, 137
children 5, 47, 74, 97, 134, 136, 155, 157 *see also* paediatrics
clinical attachments 30
clinical experience *see* experience, broadening
clinical knowledge, gathering 9–10
Cohort Study of 2006 Medical Graduates 1, 13, 60
colorectal surgery (specialty profile) 114–15
competencies 37, 50–1, 58, 82, 104, 126, 129, 134–5, 160
competition ratios 11–13, 14, 80
complaints 151, 152, 153–4
conferences 33
confidence 79
consolidation period 87–9
consultants 37, 44, 54, 65, 73, 91, 92, 96–7, 129, 133, 158, 159
contracts 90, 92–3, 126
Core Specialty Training 53, 54, 55, 56
coroners 143, 152
coupled specialties 55
court work 143, 144
cruise liners 142–3
cultural diversity 44
cultural issues, working abroad 138–9
curriculum vitae (CV)
    audits 100
    career fairs 38
    intercalated degrees 71, 72
    ROPD 22–5
    Specialty Training 101–3
    suggested information for inclusion 23–4
    volunteering 75
    working abroad 136, 137

Darzi, Lord 48–9
deaneries *see also* East Midlands Deanery; West Midlands Deanery
    appraisal 60, 62
    career support 1, 33, 34–5, 37
    competition ratios 13
    discrimination 161
    flexible training arrangements 47
    Foundation Programme 33, 61–3, 78–9, 82, 83
    inter-deanery transfers 63, 105
    medical education as preparation for work in 130
    mentoring 44
    NHS: MEE 53
    Scotland 83
    Specialty Training 101, 102, 103, 105
decisions, career 8–9
defence services 141–2
Department of Health (DoH) 41, 53, 54, 133, 159
diabetes 112, 134
'did not attend' (DNA) rates 134

direct discrimination 157–8
direct observation of procedural skills (DOPS) 59
disability 63, 134, 159–60, 161
Disability Discrimination Act 1995 and 2005 (DDA) 159, 161
disciplinary procedures 149, 151, 152, 153, 162
discrimination 44, 157–63, 168
district general hospitals 79
doctors *see also* GPs; women doctors
    career benefits 47–8, 165
    duties of 85, 157
drug misuse 76, 113, 134, 142
Duties of a Doctor 87, 157

ear, nose and throat (ENT) 111, 134
East Midlands Deanery 38
education 126, 127, 128, 129, 155 *see also* teaching; training
educational supervisors 42–3, 52, 62, 76, 89, 104, 165
electives 66–70, 137
Electives Network 68
emergency medicine 14, 75, 101, 107–8, 134, 136, 143 *see also* accident & emergency
Employment Equality (age) Regulations 2006 161
Employment Equality (religion or belief) Regulations 2003 161
Employment Equality (sexual orientation) Regulations 2003 161
endocrinology 112–13
endoscopy 114, 134
English language skills 29
epilepsy 113, 118, 134
Equality and Human Rights Commission 161
ERASMUS (European Community Action Scheme for the Mobility of University Students) 72
Estonia 72
ethnic origin, discrimination 159, 160, 161
Europe, working in 72, 137, 138, 140
European Community Action Scheme for the Mobility of University Students (ERASMUS) 72
European Health Insurance Card 138
European Working Time Directive (EWTD) 47, 52, 53, 90, 95
evidence-based medicine 48, 51, 72, 129
exams 4, 5, 54, 70, 87, 101, 103, 105, 136, 137, 155
exchange programmes, Europe 72
experience, broadening
    electives 66–70
    exchange programmes 72
    intercalated degrees 70–2
    resources 165
    student-selected components (SSCs) 64–6
    taster experiences 63, 64, 73–4, 100, 126, 127
    volunteering 75
    work experience 64, 73–4
experiences of others 4–7, 87–8, 147–8, 164 *see also* specialty profiles
extended matching questions (EMQs) 29

Flexible Careers Scheme 96
flexible training scheme 47, 95–6
flexible working 95–6, 146, 155, 157
Foreign & Commonwealth Office 67, 68, 138, 139
forensics 113, 143
Foundation Achievement of Competency Document (FACD) 60
Foundation Applicant's Handbook 81
Foundation Programme
    academic medicine 126, 127, 128, 129
    application advice 78, 81–3, 84
    appraisals 60, 62
    competition ratios 80
    deaneries 33, 61–3, 78–9, 82, 83
    devolved nations 83
    eligibility criteria 81
    Modernising Medical Careers 50–2
    Operational Framework for Foundation Training 126
    overview 58–60
    recruitment methods 53
    resources 165
    timeline for application events 83, 84
    working abroad 136, 139
Foundation schools 61–3, 78–9, 81, 82, 83
Foundation Training Programme Director (FTPD) 59
Foundation Year 1 (F1) *see also* junior doctors; pre-registration house officers (PRHOs)
    applications 78
    career advice and support 10, 37
    change of career following placement 1
    common tasks 60
    consolidation period 87, 88, 89
    experience of others 5–6, 87–8
    hours of work 90
    international graduates 29
    Modernising Medical Careers 51, 54
    overview 58–9
    pay 91
    progression to F2 63
    specialty choices 13, 14
    Tooke report recommendation 53, 54
Foundation Year 2 (F2)
    career advice and support 10
    Modernising Medical Careers 51, 54
    overview 58, 59
    pay 91
    progression from F1 63
    Tooke report recommendation 53, 54
The Foundation Years 9
France 72, 137
funding
    electives 69
    intercalated degrees 71, 72
    research 69, 126, 129

Gambia 69
gastroenterology 113–14

gay doctors 139, 159, 161
gender discrimination 158–9, 160, 162
General and Specialist Medical Practice (Education, Training and Qualifications) Order 2003 150
General Medical Council (GMC)
    discrimination 157
    Foundation Programme 58, 61, 82, 83
    Good Medical Practice 82, 85–6, 157
    guidelines 83, 85–6
    The New Doctor 59, 82
    overview 149
    registration 22, 29, 59, 82, 89, 139, 149
    Specialty Training 104
    Tomorrow's Doctors 64, 157
general practice
    academic programmes 102, 126–7
    competition ratio 13
    locum work 93, 94
    specialty profile 115–16
    training 50, 55, 56, 99
    work experience 73
general practitioners *see* GPs
Generic Standards for Training 104
genitourinary medicine 116–17
geriatrics *see* age-related medicine
Germany 72, 137
GMC *see* General Medical Council
The Gold Guide (A Reference Guide for Postgraduate Specialty Training in the UK) 96, 100, 104, 105, 127
Good Medical Practice 82, 85–6, 157
Good Mentoring Toolkit for Healthcare 45
Good Samaritan acts 151, 152
Goodenough report 58
GP registrars 91, 93
GPs (general practitioners) *see also* general practice
    earnings 91, 92
    general practice specialty profile 115–16
    premier league doctors 144
    prison doctors 142
    register 50, 51, 149
    ship's doctors 142
GPs with a special interest (GPwSI) 133–5, 166
gynaecology and obstetrics 55, 118–19, 158

harassment 157, 158, 162
health
    discrimination 159, 160, 161
    pre-employment checks 83
    shift work 94–5
    travel 68, 69, 137, 138
    work–life balance 97
healthcare assistants 74
High Quality Care for All 48–9
A High Quality Workforce 54
Higher Specialist Training 55, 56, 127
HIV (human immunodeficiency virus) 68, 117, 138, 160

homosexuality 139, 159, 161
hospital consultants 96–7, 133, 158
hospitals 75, 79
Houghton, A 13, 16, 79
hours of work
    academic medicine 127
    defence service doctors 141
    European Working Time Directive (EWTD)
      47, 52, 53, 90, 95
    flexible working 95–6, 146, 155, 157
    junior doctors 90, 91
    part-time work 47, 72–3, 74, 95, 160, 161
    shift work 94–5
Howden Medical Insurance Services 153–4
human immunodeficiency virus (HIV) 68, 117,
   138, 160

IELTS (International English Language Testing
  System) 29
illness, discrimination 159, 160, 161
Implementing Care Closer to Home 133–4, 135
'Improving Working Lives' initiative 47
income protection 154–5
indemnity insurance 69, 139, 151, 152, 153–4
India 67
indirect discrimination 158
induction periods 62
infectious diseases, working abroad 68, 138, 140
information sources 8, 9–10, 33
information technology (IT) 51
Institute for Career Guidance 35
insurance
    electives 68, 69
    income protection 154–5
    indemnity 69, 139, 151, 152, 153–4
    international doctors 30
    travel 68, 138
interactive resources 10–11, 13–20, 34, 169, 170
intercalated degrees 70–2, 129
International English Language Testing System
  (IELTS) 29
International Federation of Medical Students'
  Association (IFMSA) 72
international-graduate doctors 29–30, 44
International Medical Recruitment 139
international students 53
interview skills 25–8
Israel 69
Italy 72

job applications *see also* curriculum vitae
    electives 67, 69
    Foundation Programme 78, 81–3, 84
    international-graduate doctors 29–30
    interview skills 25–8
    record of professional development (ROPD)
      21
    rejection, dealing with 28–9
    resources 164–5
    Specialty Training 102–4

job satisfaction 48, 79
job-share 95
journalism 143, 146
journals 8, 9–10
junior doctors *see also* Foundation Year 1
    higher training posts 102
    private practice 92, 93
    working abroad 136, 139–40
    working conditions 90–1, 92
Junior Doctors' Handbook 91, 92

Keele Medical Student Career Committee 35, 38

The Lancet 10
languages 24, 29, 65, 72, 137, 140
law 71, 83, 143–4, 146, 152, 153
leadership training 55
leave entitlement *see* annual leave; maternity/
  paternity leave; study leave
lesbian doctors 139, 159, 161
libraries 8, 44, 65, 70, 129
locum work 93–4

malpractice 69, 151, 153–4 *see also* indemnity
  insurance
Malta 72
management, medical 53, 55
MARROW charity 75
maternity/paternity leave 92, 152, 161
media 123, 143, 146, 151
*The Medic's Guide to Work and Electives Around the
  World* 67
Medic's Travel 67
Medical and Defence Union of Scotland
  (MDDUS) 69, 151–2
medical defence organisations 143
Medical Defence Union (MDU) 38, 68, 69, 76, 139,
  151
Medical Education England (NHS: MEE) 53–4,
  55
Medical Forum 35, 100, 147–8, 152–3
Medical Protection Society (MPS) 38, 69, 76, 139,
  153
Medical Research Council 127, 129
medical schools
    career support 34, 35, 37–8, 53
    consolidation period 87, 88–9
    contact details 175–6
    Foundation Programme applications 82
    male entrants 158
    medical societies 36
    racism, accusations of 159
    short courses 76
    student career committees 35
    student-selected components 65
    surgical societies 35–6, 37–8
    women entrants 158
medical secretaries 74
Medical Specialties 99
Medical Success 40, 147

Medical Training Application System (MTAS) 52, 101
Medical Women's Federation 155
medicine
    competition ratio 1, 13
    core training 55
    other careers 143, 144
    revision courses 76
    specialty profiles 108, 111, 112, 119, 124, 125
    student societies 36
Medicine Publishing 10
Médecins Sans Frontières 140
MedRecruit 139
mental health 34, 61, 76, 113, 134, 142, 159
mentoring
    benefits 43–4
    definitions and main elements 41–2
    educational supervisors 42–3, 52, 62, 89, 165
    finding a mentor 44–5
    making the most of a mentor 45–6
    medical education 130
    qualities of good mentors 45
    resources 165
Merrison Report 58
mini-clinical evaluation exercise (mini-CEX) 59, 60
mini-peer assessment tool (mini-PAT) 59
Modernising Medical Careers (MMC)
    career advice 32–3, 34–5, 36–7
    career benefits 48
    career support 1, 48, 52, 99
    competition ratios 11, 13
    mentoring definition 41
    overview 50–2
    training programmes 50–2, 54, 55
    Working Group for Career Management 32, 33, 76
money see funding; pay
MTAS (Medical Training Application System) 52, 101
multi-source feedback 59
musculoskeletal medicine 134, 144
Myers-Briggs type indicator (MBTI) 16, 17, 18, 19, 160

National Health Service (NHS)
    career benefits 47–8, 165
    Darzi review 48–9
    discrimination 157
    mentoring 41
    private practice by employees 92–3
NHS Careers 35
'NHS Evidence Service' 48
NHS Jobs website 101
NHS Medical Education England (NHS: MEE) 53–4, 55
NHS Pension Scheme 92
NHS trusts
    academic medicine 126
    career support 35

performers' lists 94
    private practice by employees 92–3
National Institute for Health Research (NIHR) 127
    Coordinating Centre for Research Capacity Development 101, 126, 127, 128
National Library for Health (NLH) 8–9
National Survey of Trainees 2007 95
National Training Numbers (NTN) 104, 127
National Travel Health Network and Centre 68
Navy careers 141
nephrology (specialty profile) 117
neurology (specialty profile) 117–18
neurosurgery 55
'New Deal' 47
The New Doctor 59, 89
New Zealand 139
NHS see National Health Service
night shifts 90, 94
NIHR see National Institute for Health Research
North America 69
Northern Ireland 83, 92, 105

objective structured clinical examination (OSCE) 29
obstetrics and gynaecology 55, 118–19, 158
occupational health services 34, 161
on-call work 27, 94, 104, 144
oncology 119–20
Open University 13
Operational Framework for Foundation Training 126
ophthalmology 14, 55, 64, 109, 134
orthopaedics 11, 120–1, 134
overseas-graduate doctors 29–30, 44
overseas students 53
overseas working 67–9, 72, 92, 136–40, 166–7

paediatrics 55, 76, 121–2, 158
part-time work 47, 72–3, 74, 95, 160, 161
passports 68, 137, 138
PasTest 76, 155
pathology 13, 55, 122–3, 14, 158
patients
    discrimination 160
    interaction/relationship with 51, 59
    safety 51
pay
    academic medicine 127
    changing careers 146
    choosing rotations 79
    defence services 141
    locum work 93–4
    'New Deal' 47
    overview of salaries 90–1
    pensions 92, 146
    private practice 92–3
    resources 166
peer group activities 34, 76
pensions 92, 146
personal development plan (PDP) 60, 104

personality types
  avoiding discrimination 160
  career development toolkit 13–19
  personality toolkit 17, 34
PGMET 150
pharmaceutical industry 143, 146
PhD study 127
PLAB (Professional and Linguistic Assessments
  Board) test 29, 30
police 143, 153
portfolios 60, 104–5, 134–5
Postgraduate and Medical Education Training
  Board (PMETB) 50, 52, 61, 95, 104, 139, 149–50
postgraduate deaneries *see* deaneries
postgraduate training *see* training
Practitioners with Special Interests (PwSI) 133,
  166
premier league doctors 144
pre-registration house officers (PRHOs) 37, 58, 88,
  90 *see also* Foundation Year 1
presentation, personal 27–8
Prevention of Less Favourable Treatment
  Regulations 2000 161
primary care 19, 51, 52, 62, 74, 133
Primary Care Contracting 134
prison doctors 142, 143
private practice 92–3, 99, 112, 115, 116, 120, 151
Professional and Linguistic Assessments Board
  (PLAB) test 29, 30
psychiatry 55, 113, 143, 158
psychology services 34
psychometric testing 13, 16, 36
public health 11, 13, 55, 79, 123
published research 71, 79, 10, 130

Race Relations Act 1976 (Amendment)
  Regulations 2003 161
racism 159, 160, 161
radiology 13, 55, 123–4
recommendation letters 69
record of professional development (ROPD) 21
redundancy 92, 161
referees 24, 82
*A Reference Guide for Postgraduate Specialty
  Training in the UK (The Gold Guide)* 96, 100,
  104, 105, 127
reflection 10–11, 60, 171, 172
reflective diaries and logs 60, 76, 103, 104–5
refugee doctors 53
registration
  European Union countries 137
  General Medical Council 22, 29, 59, 82, 89,
    139, 149
  other countries 140
rejection, dealing with 28–9
religious discrimination 160, 161
research
  academic medicine 126, 127, 128, 129–30
  choosing rotations 79
  electives 69

funding 69, 126, 129
intercalated degrees 70, 71
medical education 130
publications 71, 79, 10, 130
Specialty Training prerequisite 101
student-selected components 65
volunteering 75
respiratory medicine 124–5, 134
retirement 92, 96, 152, 161
returner schemes 96, 146
revision courses 76, 87
rheumatology 125
Royal Air Force careers 141–2
Royal College of Anaesthetists 110, 173
Royal College of General Practitioners 76, 116,
  142, 173
Royal College of Obstetricians and Gynaecologists
  11, 173
Royal College of Ophthalmologists 173
Royal College of Paediatrics and Child Health 122,
  173
Royal College of Pathologists 123, 173
Royal College of Physicians 108, 109, 111, 113, 114,
  117, 118, 120, 123, 125, 142, 173
Royal College of Psychiatrists 113, 142, 173
Royal College of Radiologists 124, 174
Royal College of Surgeons of Edinburgh 115, 121,
  174
Royal College of Surgeons of England 111, 115,
  121, 159, 174
royal colleges
  career support 1, 35, 55
  contact details 173–4
  short courses 76
Royal Medical Benevolent Fund (RMBF) 47, 97–8
Royal Navy careers 141
Royal Society of Medicine (RSM) 40, 76

safety
  patients 51
  working abroad 67, 138
salaries *see* pay
SCALPEL (surgical) societies 35–6, 37–8
Scandinavia 72
Sci59 (Specialty Choice Inventory) 13, 15, 37
Scotland 61, 69, 83, 92, 105
Scottish Foundation Allocation Scheme (SFAS) 83
SCRUBS (surgical) societies 35–6, 37–8
self-employment 91, 94
senior house officers (SHOs) 59, 87–8, 159
sex discrimination 158–9, 160, 162
Sex Discrimination Act 1975 162
sexual health 116–17, 134
sexual orientation, discrimination 159, 160, 161
shadowing 73, 87–9, 100
shift work 94–5
ship's doctor 142–3
Signposting Medical Careers for Doctors 31
single best answer questions (SBAs) 20
sleep problems 94, 95

slot share 95
SORTIT 20
Specialist register 50, 51, 93
specialist registrars 91, 95, 100, 143
specialties
    competition ratios 11–13, 14, 80
    coupled and uncoupled 55, 100
    courses 75–6
    Foundation Programme 79
    GPwSI 134
    research 129–30
specialty profiles
    academic medicine 130–1
    accident and emergency 107–8
    acute medicine 108
    age-related medicine 108–9
    anaesthetics 109–10
    cardiology 110–11
    ear, nose and throat surgery 111
    endocrinology 112–13
    forensic psychiatry 113
    gastroenterology 113–14
    general and colorectal surgery 114–15
    general practice 115–16
    genitourinary medicine 116–17
    nephrology 117
    neurology 117–18
    obstetrics and gynaecology 118–19
    oncology 119–20
    orthopaedics 120–1
    paediatrics 121–2
    pathology 122–3
    public health 123
    radiology 123–4
    resources 166
    respiratory medicine 124–5
    rheumatology 125
Specialty Trainees 73
Specialty Training programme
    academic medicine 126, 127
    Annual Review of Competence Progression
      104
    application and selection 1–2, 99, 101–4
    competition ratios 11–13, 14, 80
    Core Training 53, 54, 55, 56
    devolved nations 105
    educational supervisors 104
    flexible training 96
    The Gold Guide 96, 100, 104, 105, 127
    Higher Specialist Training 55, 56, 127
    Modernising Medical Careers 50, 51
    prior experience 100
    Tooke report recommendations 53, 55, 100,
      127
    undertaking 104–5
    working abroad 139
sponsorship 69, 152, 154, 155
sports medicine 65, 144
Standing Committee on Postgraduate Medical
    Education (SCOPME) 41

stress 5, 18, 26, 37, 43, 97, 115, 129
Student BMA News 150
Student BMJ 10, 16, 150
student-selected components (SSCs) 64–6
study leave 64, 73, 93, 96, 104
substance misuse 76, 113, 134, 142
summer jobs 72–3
Summons 152
superannuation *see* pensions
supervisors, educational 42–3, 52, 62, 76, 89, 104,
    165
support4doctors 147
surgery
    competition ratios 11, 13
    female to male ratios, consultants and
      registrars 158
    general and colorectal (specialty profile)
      114–15
    personality types 19
    police surgeons 143
    revision courses 76
    student societies 35–6, 37–8
    training 55
    working abroad 136

Tanzania 67
taster experiences 63, 64, 73–4, 100, 126, 127
teaching 19, 71, 130
team assessment of behaviour (TAB) 59
teamwork 7, 17, 19, 23, 47, 51, 74, 82
third-world countries 136
Tibet 69, 136
time management 51, 130
Tomorrow's Doctors 64, 157
Tooke report (*Aspiring to Excellence*) 52–3, 54–5,
    56, 100, 127
training *see also* Foundation Programme;
    general practice – training; Specialty Training
    programme
    flexible training scheme 47, 95–6
    management and leadership 53, 55
    Modernising Medical Careers 50–2, 54, 55
    National Survey of Trainees 2007 95
    NHS Medical Education England (NHS: MEE)
      53–4, 55
    Tooke report 52–3, 54–5, 56, 100, 127
    working abroad 139
transgender doctors, discrimination 159
trauma 11, 19, 75, 101, 143
travel 67–9, 134, 136, 137–40, 144

uncoupled specialties 55, 100
United States 69, 137, 138
United States Medical Licensing Examination 137
universities *see also* medical schools
    academic medicine 126, 129
    career support 35, 37
    intercalated degrees 70–2, 129
    sports medicine 144
    volunteer work 75

University of East Anglia 65
University of London Careers Department 20

vaccinations 68
victimisation 158
visas 68, 136, 137–8
vocational training (VT) certificate 137
Voluntary Service Overseas 140
volunteer work 75, 136, 140, 144, 152

Wales 83, 92, 105
Walport posts 126–7
Wellcome Trust 69, 127
Welsh Orthopaedic Society 121
Wesleyan Medical Sickness 154–5

West Midlands Deanery 37, 39, 99, 107, 120, 130
Windmills online 16–17
women doctors 44, 96, 97, 155, 158–9
'Women in Surgical Training' initiative 159
work experience 64, 73–4
work–life balance 47, 79, 96–8, 146
working abroad 67–9, 72, 92, 136–40, 166–7
working conditions *see also* hours of work; pay
    changing careers 146
    European Working Time Directive (EWTD)
        47, 52, 53, 90, 95
    locum work 93–4
    recent improvements 90–1
    resources 166
Workstep 161